PASTORAL PRESENCE

IN

CORPORATE HEALTHCARE

IN SEARCH OF SUSTAINABILITY

By

C. JOHN MALONE

Edited by Greg Russell

Cover Design by James Ransom & Eric Malone

Graphs by Tim Malone

Foreword

It was one of those defining weeks – a few days in which dramatic events can cause sometimes abstract concepts such as the preciousness of life and the importance of ministry to hurting people to come into sharp focus. The deaths of three children in the Emergency Department, within mere days of each other, were devastating to the staff and, certainly, the families. Chaplains were called to assist the grieving. The Chaplains' healing presence and words of comfort were vital to the recovery of the staff and to the parents of those small children.

For just such times as this, Pastoral programs have been dear to me for a large part of my career. I have always believed that a pastoral presence in healthcare is a vital part of the healing process for patients, families and staff. I have witnessed and know that pastoral presence can be important to a hospital staff. I have worked in healthcare administration for more than 30 years, and Pastoral Care programs have reported to me for the majority of that time. Upon my arrival at Northwest Health System, to serve as Vice President of Human Resources for the three-hospital system, I discovered that Northwest had an active Pastoral Care program that also included a Clinical Pastoral Education (CPE) Program, led by our Director of Pastoral Care, C.J. Malone. I soon met C.J. and discovered that he not only had a great passion for his program, but he was an awesome golfer. I liked him immediately!

Within a few months, the CEO called me in and asked if I would take on the role of Associate Administrator and be administratively responsible for several other departments. Among those departments was the Pastoral Care department led by C.J. As I started to meet regularly with him, I began to realize that he was not only dedicated and caring, but he was a real pro. He had a much deeper understanding of his role as director of the department, leader of the CPE Program and as the organization Chaplain than anyone I had ever known in that role. Because of severe budget cuts, I came to C.J. one day to tell him that if we could not come up with a different delivery model for Pastoral Care, we were going to lose all of our Chaplains. C.J. went to work and delivered a new model that sustained our Pastoral Care Department and made it even better!

CEOs, CFOs, COOs and Directors of Pastoral Care all are challenged with budget pressures and "bottom line" issues. The message of this book is to convey the importance of keeping Pastoral Care sustainable in corporate-run healthcare, where it is being squeezed so tightly these days. The current healthcare environment challenges leaders to work toward understanding and compromise in the attempt to keep Pastoral Care sustainable, on one hand, and cost-effective on the other. This is the first book I have ever seen that presents unique ideas on how to sustain Pastoral Care in a corporate, for-profit or not-for-profit healthcare environment.

For those who are responsible for Pastoral Care programs, this book is the best guide on how to sustain such a program. My hope is for healthcare organizations to continue to benefit from Pastoral Care professionals. "Care" is an integral part of the term "healthcare." Yes, doctors and nurses are a vital part of that care, but healthcare depends on inter-disciplinary teams to provide complete care. Pastoral Care programs are a vital part of caring for the whole person.

Yes, death, sickness, pain and suffering will continue, but a pastoral presence provides a compassionate, healing presence that makes the journey easier.

Michael Meeks, B.S., M.B.A.

Associate Administrator/Vice President of Human Resources

Northwest Health System

Acknowledgements

Where do I begin? There are so many stories to tell of those who have impacted my life's development and professional functioning. Let me start with my parents, who are now deceased. The ways in which they reached out to help people in need continues to inspire me to reach out in love and kindness to those who are hurting and to stand up for social-justice issues. My children have been a constant comfort and encouragement to me over the years, as I have attempted to fulfill my parenting role. My wife Donise, who in 1973 directed our junior class play in high school, (in which I played a role) is a godsend, and there was no way to know at that time where life would lead us, but 2009 changed our worlds.

It's important that I thank my CPE Supervisors William DeLong, John Valentino and William "Ed" Outlaw who mentored me through the CPE Supervisory process, starting with ACPE and continuing on to Diplomate certification in CPE Supervision with the College of Pastoral Supervision and Psychotherapy. Special thanks to Mike Meeks, my former boss, who agreed to write the foreword to this book, and to all those who helped edit what was written. Special thanks to all the caring and compassionate CEOs, CFOs, CNOs, nurses and ancillary staff and auxiliary volunteers with whom I have worked in the past. Most importantly, I thank God for placing a passion within me to reach out to people who are hurting and in need of professional Pastoral Care and presence. I have listened to many of their stories, and I hope they can spend a few moments reading about my story, as it unfolds in the following pages.

Introduction

Pastoral Care is my calling and my passion. My objective in writing this volume is to help those on the front lines in corporate-run healthcare to position Pastoral Care as a valued, integral and "sustainable" part of the healthcare delivery system, even as the new face of healthcare continues to emerge in the decades to come. How do Pastoral Care services mesh with corporate healthcare? How do Pastoral Care providers function in a healthcare environment driven by the "bottom line"? How does Pastoral Care affect the culture of corporate healthcare? What are some of the current trends related to Pastoral Care services in corporate healthcare? Should a hospital rely solely on volunteers to meet the religious and spiritual needs of its patients, visitors and employees? Should Pastoral Care duties be relegated to other hospital staff? These and other poignant questions will be addressed in this book.

In these tough economic times, healthcare is being treated as a commodity and traded on Wall Street. And healthcare corporations, in their quest to grow their "bottom lines," swallow staff like a hungry person devouring a good chicken dinner. My hope is that this book will stimulate creative thought and action to sustain a fertile ministry field and offer sound direction to our corporate leaders, Directors of Pastoral Care, care providers and staff who are affected by the rampant corporate acquisitions and massive changes facing America's healthcare delivery system. My desire is that this book will serve as a catalyst that will help pastoral presence solidify its position and strengthen its voice in the corporate-controlled healthcare environment.

When a hospital or healthcare system is acquired by a healthcare corporation, and the hospital or healthcare system being acquired has an active Pastoral Care department, the purchasing entity has inherited a valuable asset. As you will learn in this book, trained Pastoral Care providers working diligently (often behind the scenes) to uphold the culture, mission, vision and values of the hospital or healthcare system they serve, often are an overlooked stabilizing element. Yet, a professional Pastoral Care provider will tell you that it's not about them – it's all about the patient. This is a dynamic perspective that so many healthcare workers seem to have forgotten. The patient is the customer, and a professional Pastoral Care provider knows how to empower patients to tell their own stories, knowing full well that in so doing, a catharsis is experienced, resulting in the patient being more willing to be actively involved in the plan for their care.

Imagine if every inter-disciplinary team player were "on the same page" as the patient and how that would affect healing and the patient's length of stay. Not only do Pastoral Care providers listen to a patient's story and what's behind it, they know that the overall benefit of providing quality Pastoral Care services is that HCAHPS (Hospital Consumer Assessment of Healthcare Providers and Systems) scores will rise, and everyone caring for the patient will benefit. An empowered patient is an active participant in their own care.

For those who are in healthcare settings in which Pastoral Care services are long-standing and greatly appreciated but would like to do more to reach out to their community clergy, Eucharistic ministers, Stephen leaders, spiritual advisers and first-responders with some quality Pastoral Care training, this book contains some great suggestions.

Perhaps you work for a not-for-profit hospital or healthcare system that is about to be purchased by a for-profit entity. Or maybe you work at a for-profit hospital or healthcare system that has been acquired before and is being sold again. In corporate healthcare, there are times when hospitals are sold and staff members find themselves caught in the middle. It becomes a daunting task for staff to relax as changes take place all around them at an unprecedented rate. Trusting new owners, when employees see staff being reduced to cut costs, is difficult at best. I have found a great deal of opportunity for Pastoral Care providers to assist Administration, mid-level managers, employees and others during corporate acquisitions. Included in chapter four is a diagram that identifies many of the common phases that occur during acquisitions and the process of gaining a new identity. My personal experience, having been through a few acquisitions over the years, has aided me in designing this diagram, identifying dominate behaviors in each phase and providing some personal insight for Pastoral Care providers who may be going through an acquisition themselves.

This book is not written to be a scathing review of corporate-run healthcare's treatment of Pastoral Care services as much as it is to be a creative challenge extended to Pastoral Care providers in a cost-conscious healthcare environment to recognize trends and explore creative ways to make their services cost-effective, sustainable and progressive. That being said, this book will not be devoid of implied or explicit comments about corporate CEOs and administrators, based on my personal experiences and observations. However, if such comments are stated, they will be balanced with challenges to Pastoral Care providers as well.

As I was growing up, my mother always reminded me that there were two sides to every story. In my personal and professional life, I have tried to remain open-minded and look at both perspectives as I encounter challenging issues. That philosophy carries over into the debate between for-profit and not-for-profit healthcare. It is my goal to refrain from this debate in general and focus more specifically on my personal experiences with for-profit healthcare systems and some of the effects their actions have had on mid-level management, in particular.

It has been my observation over the past 14 years in both corporate-run healthcare and non-profit or religious-based hospitals and healthcare systems that many Directors of Pastoral Care, Clinical Pastoral Education (CPE) Supervisors and Pastoral Care providers or staff Chaplains have allowed themselves to become complacent and even lose focus as they continue to walk the halls of their hospital or healthcare system. Instead of engaging their whole healthcare environment, they find comfort and safety in serving a narrowly defined group and rarely interacting with their CEO, administrators, corporate leadership, physicians and mid-level management. To those who are feeling the effects of "burn-out," and complacency, my hope is that this book will open their eyes to the challenges and opportunities that await them, if they are willing to blow on the embers.

For Pastoral Care services to experience ongoing presence and sustainability in corporate-run healthcare, directors of Pastoral Care departments and Clinical Pastoral Education programs will need to be more creative at re-framing and realigning their services. Challenging economic times and the elimination of jobs in Pastoral Care have quickly taught us that we are facing a new day. While quality Pastoral Care services certainly benefit patients, family members, employees, physician satisfaction scores and good relations with area clergy, in corporate healthcare, profitability and the "bottom line" rules the day.

People who have worked in healthcare for very long know that "do more with less" has become the mantra – even when it comes to staffing. Corporate healthcare is driven to stay on the leading edge, with new products, procedures and service lines, all delivered with the highest possible level of quality and expediency. The purpose of this focus on the "latest and greatest" is to enhance revenue and profitability. It is my belief that Pastoral Care departments should be doing the same thing. We will review some trends in healthcare and look at ways Pastoral Care can be more cost-effective.

Venturing out into a "free-standing" entity for Pastoral Care delivery has been an interesting personal journey, so I have shared some of that exciting and challenging adventure within these pages. I also have included a straight-forward address to healthcare CEOs, regarding the importance of Pastoral Care Services and factors that should be weighed when making decisions related to their future.

Chapter One - My Story

So how did I get into Chaplaincy, anyway? As I look back at significant events in my life that have impacted me deeply, I am able to see how each one, in its own unique way, has connected with others to create a pathway to my becoming a Pastoral Care provider and Clinical Pastoral Education supervisor.

My story, though unique to me, is certainly not as moving as many of the other stories that I have listened to from scores of patients, staff, physicians and parishioners over the years. In many of those stories, there seemed to be a thread that has connected a string of life events and experiences and has led them to where they are today. Yet, the question is still a valid one: What causes a person to choose a particular profession? It is quite revealing as one looks at early life experiences and how they impact a person, challenging them to explore a deeper understanding not only of the event itself, but also of the dynamics surrounding it. Why did this happen to me? What is the life purpose behind it? How can I use my experiences to help others? Before you know it, the desire to find answers draws a person into a specific professional area, in which the focus is to be present for others who have similar questions about life experiences. At a recent Pastoral Care seminar hosted by Northwest Clinical Pastoral Institute, speaker Robert C. Dykstra (1) remarked that if a person can't remember much about his or her childhood, it was probably a pretty normal childhood. On the other hand, he noted, people who have abusive, chaotic and traumatic experiences in their upbringing usually are scarred for life. Such persons will need to go back to do some significant work in their quest for understanding and healing. The more work they do back there, the less often they will need to revisit the past.

Have you ever thought about the role genetics play in behavior, risk-taking or even in choosing a specific profession? In a National Children's Study (2) that is currently being conducted throughout America (and which is sponsored by the National Institutes of Health), one of the many areas of impact being explored are genetic factors. In the early 1990s, I began researching our family genealogy and discovered that William Copege, (Coppedge), an ancestor of mine, was Chaplain at Queens College at Oxford University in 1542, under Queen Katherine Parr. (3) Perhaps his experience made a genetic imprint that found its way through the generations and planted a love of Chaplaincy in me. No matter if it is genetically imprinted, experientially extrapolated or driven in some other manner, the reason a person chooses a specific profession is interesting to explore. Knowing from where we have come and embracing our experiences makes us a more complete individual.

In 1967, physicians could not save my little brother, Stephen, from dying of double pneumonia and a weak heart. I was just 11 years old, but, I can still remember having him in our living room area, with a sheet draped over his crib to create a vapor tent. Seeing the vapors pumped into the cavity where he lay and watching his little chest rise and fall made me wonder what was going on inside his body. Stephen was the youngest in our sibling group, and we all loved him very much. On the Saturday before his death, another of my brothers and I were rough-housing in the living room where he lay in his vapor tent. I will never forget our father telling us that we should be praying for our little brother instead of horsing around. Those words shot through me like a bolt of lightning and made an indelible mark on me because I sensed that my father was deeply concerned. It wasn't until later on in life, after I had children of my own, that I could understand to some degree the stress that my parents were experiencing in those sensitive moments as Stephen teetered between life and death – caught between two worlds.

Early the next morning, Stephen took a turn for the worse, and the physician on call at a small rural hospital in Central Illinois was paged. In spite of his efforts and the efforts of the nursing staff to save him, Stephen died. My mother often told us that she actually saw his spirit leave his body and float out the window. Etched in my memory is that Sunday morning in Sunday School class, when around 9:50 a.m., my teacher told me that Stephen had died. The pencil I was holding fell from my hand, and I was launched into a dimension of life I had never known before.

Later on, my parents learned that the physician who attended to Stephen had been at a party the night before and was obviously still feeling the effects. My mother said she could smell alcohol on his breath and noticed that his behavior and demeanor was affected. The doctor was angry with my mother for not bringing Stephen in sooner, even though she had just taken him in on Friday. Many times throughout the years, my parents would re-live that experience with us and conclude by saying that there probably was nothing the physician could have done to save his life. That realization is probably what kept my parents from filing an incident report against the doctor or taking legal action, which also would have been in conflict with their beliefs. No Chaplain was present to help my parents enter the grief process, and to this day, I don't know if they let my mother hold Stephen and rock him after he died. I know how important that is to a mother's closure work following the loss of a child. Now, I often serve as a mother's advocate, when a criminal investigation is unfolding.

My father felt he needed to be strong for our mother and the eight remaining children, plus the congregation he was leading at that time. He carried his unresolved grief for years to come. My mother would visit Stephen's grave every day, and I can remember my younger siblings and I going along with her on many occasions. Out of concern for my mother's well-being, my father thought it best to search for another church to pastor, in hopes that a change in location would help with my mother's grief. He had no training in the stages of grief, and interrupting my mother's grief process directed her grief work inward for years. She found herself 400 miles away from the grave. As a result, her normal impact stage shifted to unresolved/complicated grief, which took her more than 30 years to process. I will never forget that visit to my parents' home nearly 30 years after Stephen's death. I entered the guest bedroom, only to find his picture and bronzed shoes sitting on the dresser. I opened that top dresser drawer and gazed once again at the neatly folded clothes that Stephen once wore that mom had kept tucked away. I knew in that moment that her grief work had reached a milestone. She was finally embracing her deep loss and celebrating a life that had meant so much to her and to all of us.

Our family moved from Hillsboro, Ill., to Boone, Iowa, in the summer of 1967, which created not only a change in my mother's grief processing but some excitement for our family as a whole. Moving to another state, attending a new school and meeting new friends seemed to help distract us from the pain of the past couple of years. This was my fifth-grade year, and I had mentioned to my family that I wanted to be a physician. In retrospect, I am sure the events of Stephen's death had a large part to play in that declaration. However, I definitely knew that helping others in the midst of deep emotional pain was going to play a major role in my life, but I didn't know just how involved I would be with those who were hurting.

All fifth-grade students in the State of Iowa were required to take the Iowa Standardized Aptitude test. Several weeks later, when the teacher opened the door between the classrooms A & B to announce results, I was totally surprised to learn that I had scored the highest out of both classes. The humiliating part that soon followed was when my teacher asked me how I had cheated on the test. Since I was in the "B" class and did not normally function on that level, she was in a quandary in figuring this one out. Since that experience, I have had some difficulty with test anxiety.

What I find ironic, as I look back on my pathways, is that instead of becoming a physician to correct an injustice or lack of professional attention in the case of my brother, Stephen, I have become a Chaplain to physicians. I work with many physicians and medical staff who share with me, on a personal and professional level, the challenges they encounter as they give of themselves to bring healing to others. Many times, I have sat with physicians who are wracked with self-doubt, wondering what they could have done differently to save a life. No doubt, the physician who was present for my brother, Stephen, revisited that event many times over. Not only do I have occasion to see the inside of human hearts, brains and body cavities, but I have lived enough of life to identify with many of the inner struggles that people experience. The skills and experiences I have acquired help me do so without taking their struggle on as my own. My role as a Chaplain, Director of Pastoral Care and Executive Director of a Clinical Pastoral Education Institute is not a substitute in any way for not becoming a physician. Rather, it is God's pathway, taking me into a fulfilling life of professional, caring service, which is what I love to do but something that I never could have imagined as a fifth-grader.

Pastoral Care professionals must have the capacity and desire to embrace their past experiences in order to find a deeper meaning for life now and in the future. Those who spend the time and energy needed to process past hurts, abuses, traumas and life-changing experiences are unique individuals. When they tap into that inner spiritual ability they can transcend that which could have ensnared them in the past. Without that discovery, their future, at best, would be consumed by the past. When a person who has experienced such a past weaves together the "why's and "what fur's of their life experiences into usable material, they then can make sense of their life and help others as well. As they are

20

present with others, they may pull something from their basket to be used in a sacred moment, without diminishing the processing of those who are hurting.

My early years in the ministry held little indication that I would wind up spending so much of my career helping hurting people in hospitals, let alone training others to do so. After planting an inter-denominational community church in Michigan, moving on to a ministry team in Arkansas at an inter-denominational community church and experiencing many ministry and personal events in-between, I was several years into ministry before I first heard of Clinical Pastoral Education. I was curious from the onset, and it didn't take long for me to realize that clinical training was for me. Never had I experienced such freedom in giving and receiving feedback. Nor had I ever experienced someone holding up a mirror for me, so I could see myself and my ministry as others do. Knowing that there were scores of other ministers out there who did not know about CPE and its benefits drew me into supervision. This new-found ministry niche was a place where I could engage willing ministry servants who had suffered life wounds and be present for them as they found the recovery and healing they needed to make possible their reconnection with ministry that had deeper purpose and meaning. Over the years, I have supervised many wounded souls who were willing to trust a process and find the healing balm they needed.

It is truly an honor to walk alongside those who have been wounded by life and ministry and watch them (perhaps for the very first time) experience a K'hila K'dosha (Holy Community) of like-minded peers, holding up the mirror for each other in order to see themselves in a healing perspective. To see wholeness and joy return to these people in their journey of discovery is priceless. Then, to see them utilize the art of Pastoral Care by being present for others in need, without having their past abuses, negative experiences or religious agenda interfere is truly remarkable. For me, the challenge is to see a student put theory and practice together in a practical way that benefits a person in need.

Back in the fifth grade, I never could have imagined owning the distinct honor of coordinating a Biomedical Ethics Committee for a three-hospital system, coordinating an Institutional Review Board, serving on many committees that look closely at honoring patient rights and assess how a hospital honors, respects and serves them in their time of need. Neither could I have imagined experiencing and training interns to liaison with patients who are having coronary artery bypass graft surgery, craniotomies and other major, life-saving surgeries. Nor could I have envisioned serving as a liaison between a surgery team and a family whose members are experiencing high anxiety and clinging to hope, keeping them updated and helping them navigate this very emotional experience. This role, however, is one that is very much appreciated by family members. That's the personal caring service that keeps them returning for more quality care.

The entire Pastoral Care Department (from director to interns) make ourselves available for every event that may benefit from pastoral presence. Being an inter-disciplinary team player in a clinical environment has unique benefits. Team members draw from each other and collectively work to understand each patient as a whole person and treat him or her with care and kindness, as they seek healing of body, soul and mind. It has been said many times and in many ways: "If you love your work, you will never work a day in your life." All the Clinical Pastoral Education interns who pass through Northwest Clinical Pastoral Education Institute are reminded that when they apply the skills required in the art of Pastoral Care and become skilled in the art itself, Chaplaincy is not work. An intern experiences an inner transformation when he or she truly grasps the art of Pastoral Care and moves from doing Pastoral Care to being present for those who are in pain – going where they need to go. Allowing the patient to do his or her own work is vital to spiritual healing.

Chaplaincy and Clinical Pastoral Education has become a specialized ministry focus of mine for many years. The focus for the rest of my professional career as a Pastoral Care provider is to keep it sustainable for all those who have benefited from good Pastoral Care and presence in the past and those who require it now and in the future.

Looking back now, with the benefit of 30 years of hindsight, I can clearly see the path that has led me to this healing ministry. I truly view my work as a calling. Some callings are overt. Some people know from an early age what they are destined to do. But most stories, I believe, are like mine. As we live our lives, we are scarred and/or molded by the events that unfold, and perhaps we are unaware that these milestones are guiding us to embrace a particular vocation or passion, but that is exactly where they are leading us. If we are fortunate, they direct us to a calling that will enable us to uplift and equip others to minister in their own right. I am blessed on all counts, and I love what I am called to do.

Chapter Two – Changes & Trends

As we all know, healthcare in America is going through myriad changes. Current healthcare reforms and their legal challenges leave the majority of us wondering what healthcare will look like in the next decade. Some of those changes are a direct result of legislation, and others are due to the ever-changing economic and healthcare insurance landscapes. Healthcare cannot ship its hospitals out of the country and then sell its product and services back to the American consumer, as has happened in many other industries. In the past few years, it has become somewhat fashionable, in some circles, to visit other countries for the express purpose of undergoing specialized medical procedures, which are offered at a cost much lower than in the United States. These specialized procedures (offered by foreign physicians, many of whom have been trained in American hospitals) are accompanied by five-star accommodations and a recuperation vacation to follow. And we have heard of the tainted drugs (produced in foreign countries) that have affected consumers in our country.

Meanwhile, medical centers in community after community throughout the United States vie to serve healthcare needs and to build a positive reputation, so consumers will trust in their services and return for their future healthcare needs. Competition is alive in American healthcare.

This creative tension to offer quality healthcare and patient services profitably is felt by for-profit and not-for-profit entities alike. As a Pastoral Care provider, it has placed a drive in me to empower the patient and to become an advocate in his or her quest to receive the best care and services we have to offer. When I receive complaints from patients about costly healthcare, I agree and inwardly vow to do my part to keep the cost of our services affordable, while at the same time keeping the healthcare system's bottom line healthy. If the hospital doors close, patients are more vulnerable, and jobs are lost. It is important for me to remind myself often that I am an active member of the whole process from start to finish; from the moment a patient walks through the doors, until they are discharged. Even as I meet former patients out in the community, I continue to be a key part of the experience they had in our healthcare system. If that experience was less than they expected, I will be a catalyst in service recovery. Like ministry, healthcare is about relationships.

In October 2009, while enjoying the morning meal at a bed-and-breakfast on Montmartre in Paris, my wife and I were at the table with two other couples – one from Holland and the other from the United Kingdom. At that time, healthcare was a hot topic in America, and all the debate about the status of healthcare in America was being discussed not only at home but virtually around the world. It was a good opportunity for me to get another perspective, so I asked, "What do you think of healthcare in America?" They wondered what all the fuss was about and then went on to explain how the healthcare system worked in their countries and turned the question back to us by asking, "Why is it such an issue for Americans?" As we ate a delicious breakfast from the table of a Frenchman and his Moroccan wife, our conversation boiled down to the issue of entitlement for citizenry. It was quite revealing how socialized medicine and entitlement has cast such a long shadow. However, that is a debate that will continue to go on in America for many years to come.

Your latest trip to the hospital, like the receipt from your most recent trip to the local Gas Station, reveals the fact that healthcare services, like the cost of fuel at the pump, is becoming more and more expensive. Rarely do we see cost reductions. The price of products and services are skyrocketing. "Self-pay" turns into "no pay" as bills go uncollected and are charged off as much as the law allows. Healthcare systems are becoming as creative as possible to collect fees up front. High material and labor costs, along with length-of-stay debates, go back and forth between hospital case managers, physicians and insurance companies like a Ping-Pong ball in a world-class table tennis match.

In an attempt to provide affordable healthcare to the consumer, Pastoral Care departments need to become discretionary with the services they provide and use wisdom as they deliver their services. In his book "Contract Pastoral Care and Education – The Trend of the Future," Larry VenderCreek said, (4) institutional Pastoral Care and education are heavily dependent upon the structure of the healthcare system, and that system is changing in ways that often are not very friendly. Many departments are being reduced in size, and Chaplains have lost their jobs. In medical centers (perhaps many), concern and pessimism regarding the future of institutional ministry is the order of the day. That was in 1999, and more than a decade later, that assessment still is apropos. Like any other industry, healthcare is being challenged to run a tight ship to protect jobs and provide needed services. Pastoral Care needs to do the same, and now is the time to begin.

In the midst of this changing healthcare landscape, the Studer Group (5) and others have been hard at work projecting a culture whose objective is to keep up with changes and put patient care back as the focal point where it must be in order for patients to return for more of our healthcare. Hardwiring some basic patient-care principles has helped raise patient satisfaction scores. However, increased demands on staff and hospitals, in the form of corporate mandates and productivity expectations is another dynamic to be addressed. Mid-level managers who feel supported by their administrators will, in turn, have productive staffs. When a staff is spread much too thin, its members can easily become tired and disillusioned. Who addresses this dynamic in your hospital or healthcare system? How is staff shored up during these times? If nothing is being done at present, it will reflect in employee surveys and production levels. There are many people on the front lines of healthcare delivery who deserve to have someone walking alongside them as they struggle to provide the best care they can for those who are hurting.

Most Pastoral Care departments in corporate healthcare do not provide billable services that defray the cost of their services. If there is no financial justification for offering Pastoral Care, the medical center or healthcare system must shoulder that cost and assess how that service justifies its existence. When we look at satisfaction scores from patients, staff and physicians and include the community's perception of pastoral presence to those in need, the presence of a Pastoral Care department certainly is a valued asset.

The new face of healthcare, which continues to emerge, Medicare/Medicaid reimbursement levels are being tied more closely to patient HCAHPS scores. The HCAHPS survey (6) is the first national, standardized, publicly reported quantification of patient opinions, elements of their satisfaction with the care received and their evaluation of the environment in which it was delivered. HCAHPS is the new driving force in healthcare quality improvement, and may become a deciding factor for patients as they choose a medical center or healthcare system. It is certainly my belief that Pastoral Care Providers can make a significant difference in impacting those scores. In the midst of the changes and trends in healthcare, Pastoral Care should find acceptance and sustainability. We also will discuss the benefits of Pastoral Care when corporate acquisitions occur and mandate come rolling down to mid-level management and nursing staff.

Trends

Like a mosaic, when all the pieces are placed together and the observer steps back the proper distance, the many parts blend together to reveal the "bigger picture," which becomes clear in a broader perspective. In a recent trip to Precious Moments Chapel in Carthage, Mo., my wife and I saw a picture of Samuel Butcher stepping back to view his painted version of "Hallelujah Square," which I thought was simply magnificent. After hours of detailed painting, a step back gives new perspective. Often, it is difficult, in a fast-paced corporate setting, for a Director of Pastoral Care who is intent on providing quality spiritual care and counsel around the clock, to pause, step back and allow new perspectives to emerge. A large part of this book is a personal challenge to do that very thing.

I've made mental notes of the significant changes and some minor ones that our healthcare system has experienced over the years. Stepping back and reflecting on those changes has helped me see the emerging picture and gain a new perspective before stepping back into the painting mode once again. My encouragement to Directors of Pastoral Care in corporate settings is to make note of how your environment is changing around you. Some changes are subtle, while others are swift and blatant. Over time, those changes will blend together to provide a clear visual of an emerging new reality. As you process changes in your setting, a fresh new picture will emerge. Your challenge will be to embrace it or move on.

There have been many changes in our healthcare system over the past decade. We simply are not the same as we once were. Some things have gotten better and some have worsened. Changes have come from the effect of economic, environmental, corporate or political realities, while others are the effect of leadership decisions. As I step back to observe healthcare today, some corporate brush strokes are certainly identifiable. For art critics, getting into the mind of the artist is always a challenge. Artists know that every stroke of the brush has meaning and can become identifiable. This list of trends is by no means comprehensive, and different people's experiences may offer many more. However, this list may stimulate some personal observations and may they help prompt an important question: "What is driving these trends?"

Elimination of Pastoral Care programs

Unless a Pastoral Care department offers creative and cost-effective ways to positively impact the "bottom line," it runs a great risk of cuts and possible elimination. The recent steep economic downturn has made it even more clear that "working smart" and exploring new and effective ways of delivering Pastoral Care is the order of the day.

In an economic impact report provided by the American Hospital Association in the fall of 2010, (7) the percentage of hospitals making changes to weather the economic storm was high. Here are a few "factoids" from that revealing report:

- A total of 76 percent of hospitals had cut administrative costs.
- A surprising 73 percent had delayed capital investments.
- More than half (53 percent) had reduced staff.
- One quarter had cut services.
- About 3 percent had merged with another facility/entity.
- Approximately 24 percent had made other changes.

Perhaps the most telling statistics, however, are that since the start of the recession in 2008:

- A startling 98 percent of hospitals have not restored eliminated or reduced services or programs.
- A full 89 percent have not added back staff or increased hours.
- Up to 67 percent have continued to freeze capital projects.

The recession was not supposed to hit healthcare as hard as other sectors of our economy, but according to this data, it has, and hospitals have made some deep cuts. Hopefully, those reductions have not occurred merely to meet budget projections, or worse, to meet bonus criteria for healthcare executives.

When the economy is soft, many variables become less predictable. The decision to eliminate Pastoral Care services and staff Chaplains is an option placed on the table more often than those of us who depend upon Pastoral Care for our livelihoods care to know. During challenging economic times, administrators and CFOs look seriously at cutting staff in non-clinical departments, and Pastoral Care services become an easy target. Doing more with less is the end result for those who survive the cuts.

Reduction in Pastoral Care staff

It is expected that Pastoral Care departments in corporate-run healthcare adjust their services to provide coverage with fewer staff. Professional Pastoral Care organizations that certify Chaplains have created a patient/Chaplain matrix, but this formula often goes by the wayside when a corporate "bottom line" is threatened. (8) Many sacrifices are made in response to financial pressures, and that trend is not likely to change anytime soon.

When a Pastoral Care position has been eliminated, others in the department must step up to fill the void. The department director must address the reduction with his or her remaining staff, and a plan to provide the coverage needed must be explained and implemented. It is important that time be given for the remaining staff to process the loss and make their critical adjustments, personally and professionally. Over the course of a decade, my staff went from four FTEs, down to one – myself. CPE student interns fulfill their clinical training/practice requirements by providing coverage, under my supervision, and contract Chaplains (compensated from an outside source) are utilized as well. I will discuss this in greater detail later. When nursing staff hear of Pastoral Care reductions, they usually are the first to voice their opinions, since they are on the front lines of care and see the immediate impact of pastoral presence on patients, family and staff. As a Pastoral Care director, I allowed time for staff nurses to vent and process such losses. When pastoral care staff reductions occur, the Director of Pastoral Care should stay focused and start thinking "outside the box." The people who are deciding to make cuts will have little or no insight into the full scope of a Pastoral Care staff person's responsibilities. Remaining staff, if any are left, must work "smarter." Staff members who cannot make the adjustment are left to the wastelands. A good explanation from Administration to the Pastoral Care director as to why the cuts are necessary is vital to morale. If such a rationale is not provided, the Director should explain the forces behind the cuts as best he or she can. Otherwise, the reason for the reductions is left to employees' imaginations and the "rumor mill."

As medical centers and healthcare systems continue to cut Pastoral Care positions, it is interesting to note that there are other opportunities becoming available for Pastoral Care providers. A positive glimmer on the horizon is that, with the aging "Baby Boomer" generation, healthcare systems, nursing homes and hospice organizations will find themselves in need of pastoral presence more than ever. Also, many "Baby Boomers" are becoming "Holy Enrollers," returning to seminaries and entering ministry as a second career. It is also interesting to note that industry is utilizing Chaplains for their Employee Assistance Programs (as counselors) and as Job Coaches. A number of major corporations in our area, such as Tyson and Simmons Foods, utilize the presence of a Chaplain in their production plants, and those types of opportunities are expected to grow.

Pastoral Care Directors utilizing volunteer community clergy

Directors of Pastoral Care in corporate-run healthcare settings throughout America are being instructed by their Administrations to utilize local clergy to meet Pastoral Care needs as they arise. This trend is most commonly found in smaller to mid-sized rural hospitals, but the practice is creeping into larger metropolitan areas as well. Years ago, many people in rural areas were connected with local churches and had access to a pastor's care. But it is worth noting that in our society today, more and more people are without a church affinity. Those individuals also deserve

34

Pastoral Care and Presence during crisis situations in their lives if they request it.

Since not-for-profit hospitals affiliated with faith-based organizations have experienced a nominal degree of effectiveness with this local clergy volunteer model, some for-profit systems assume that it is a viable, cost-saving option for them. While utilizing local clergy to do the work of an employed Pastoral Care team may not be violating any fair labor laws per se, the standard seems to be clear that it should not be done solely for financial reasons [FLSA 29 U.S.C. 203 (c) and 29 U.S.C 201 et. Seq.]. The intent of this action should be looked at very closely. In most cases, I have discovered it boils down to a way to cut costs. My personal angst about this practice is that those who suggest it rarely suggest similar tactics be employed in their own roles. I am tempted to ask, "Where are the volunteer Administrators?" Surely there are executives from other industries or retired hospital administrators in the community who could step in and deliver a level of service approximate to that achieved by the current paid Administration – only for free. And I won't even ask about the volunteer heart surgeons. The careful reader probably will detect a tinge of sarcasm in my tone. The simple reality is that healthcare administrators often do not see the "disconnect" between what they "preach" and what they practice, when it comes to the subject of substituting volunteers in place of professionals. And on the other side of the coin, I'm sure administrators would not take on additional work, outside of their paying jobs, unless they were paid as a consultant. Yet, under this volunteer clergy model, this is exactly what they are asking of them while they have their own congregations to shepherd.

These volunteer clergy are expected to be present for traumas, deaths and mass-casualty events and to possess the skills and knowledge necessary to minister in a healthcare setting, to be present for those in need … at all hours of the night and day. If local volunteer clergy are utilized, they should never be expected to shoulder the cost of the specialized training required to equip them to serve effectively in a healthcare setting. That cost should be borne by the healthcare organizations that benefit from their volunteered services. Furthermore, I would recommend that special acts of appreciation for clergy volunteers be made by the hospital or healthcare system. What other professional discipline offers its services for free?

The effectiveness and success of this model depends on the availability of local clergy to volunteer their time and dedicate themselves to required training in crisis intervention, pastoral presence, inter-disciplinary functioning, family systems, cultural dynamics and several other dimensions of Pastoral Care. Most engaged community clergy do not have available time to volunteer. A point to also remember is that while some community clergy classify themselves as non-denominational or inter-denominational, most are aligned with a mainstream denomination. Due to the fact that they are not integrated as a part of the hospital staff, few volunteer clergy follow up with staff or physicians for defusing or debriefing after a crisis event. Some patients, family and staff may demonstrate resistance when a volunteer clergy of a denomination or faith group that is different from their own responds to their need.   And in rural communities, when a trauma involves a congregation member or parishioner of the volunteer clergy on call, he or she may be just as impacted by the event as the family. In such an event, established self-care protocol should dictate that a backup volunteer clergy be called, because the patient's clergy may find himself or herself in need of Pastoral Care.

In assessing this model, my purpose is not to cast aspersions on it but to provide real issues for consideration. In doing so, I want to acknowledge that there are effective all-volunteer clergy programs in existence. In those programs, of which I have been a part in the past, the volunteer clergy person focuses on providing their services in times of death and major trauma cases. The success and effectiveness of this model depends on the availability and willingness of local clergy and retired ministers to volunteer their time. The director to whom they report must draw clear boundaries and screen volunteers, so not just anyone who calls himself or herself a minister will have access to patients. There are certainly many things to consider before utilizing local clergy in a medical center.

Many mega churches have their own Pastoral Care or Eucharistic teams that utilize retired ministers and other trained Pastoral Care providers. They have become effective care providers for their congregants. Directors of Pastoral Care can be helpful in facilitating their access to members in accordance with the Healthcare Insurance Portability and Accountability Act (HIPAA) and its privacy requirements and departmental protocols.

In hospitals throughout rural America and in some mid-sized urban settings in which hospitals do not have paid Chaplains or Directors of Pastoral Care, the hospital Auxiliary Director or Volunteer Coordinator takes over the responsibility of scheduling Pastoral Care coverage and services through local clergy and retired ministers. They recruit them and do their best to train them in spiritual and cultural assessments, crisis intervention, clinical matters and hospital protocol. At times they will locate a person who has experience in Pastoral Care to do the training for them. In order to properly respond to patients' wishes (and to achieve accreditation by the Joint Commission), a hospital must have a "qualified person" to perform spiritual assessments and address the cultural and religious needs of patients. The question is how should "qualified person" be interpreted? The volunteer clergy model is found more often than one might imagine and it's anyone's guess as to how qualified those clergy are in assessing age specific spiritual care.

A great challenge for those in charge of this program is when local clergy cannot fill coverage gaps and there are no pastoral care staff, who covers the pastoral care need? This model also assumes that local clergy are effective Pastoral Care providers which is often not the case. As stated previously, many area clergy lack professional training in Pastoral Care and carry their own theological or denominational agenda into the visit with them. As I have seen time and again, clergy encounter situations for which they are ill-equipped and find themselves in need of defusing. They could certainly benefit from more clinical training.

As America becomes more acculturated, even smaller rural communities are seeing a broader spectrum of faith groups. Mainline denominations are waning. Relying on a Christian minister who has very little formal and clinical training as to how to meet the spiritual needs of a Muslim patient in their time of crisis may not be what the Joint Commission has in mind, when it comes to a "qualified person" for addressing patients' religious and cultural needs.

In this model, the Auxiliary Director or Volunteer Coordinator is entrusted with the responsibility to coordinate volunteer clergy and/or contact the patient's clergy for spiritual care, if requested to do so by the patient or family. It's interesting to note that more and more patients do not have a church affinity, so healthcare organizations must formulate plans as to how to address these patients' spiritual and religious needs. For those after-hours and weekend trauma events, the House Supervisor (this person is a nurse who is charged with overseeing the hospital's patient-care operations after normal business hours) should be trained to make those calls to the on-call clergy or the patient's clergyperson. Most house supervisors lack formal theological or clinical pastoral training themselves and are ill-prepared to provide spiritual or pastoral care to patients and their family if clergy cannot be reached.

Not to be redundant here, but in order to meet the Joint Commission RI standard for assessing the patient's spiritual or religious needs, one should have the appropriate training to do so. For me, this means that the person who assesses a patient's spiritual need should have appropriate theological, cultural, religious or spiritual training to do a complete psycho-social-spiritual-religious assessment. The all-volunteer clergy model, as cost-saving as it may appear to be, presents major concerns. Without pastoral presence on staff, employees do not have someone they can go to when they need to defuse or decompress. Clinical staff rarely have rapport with the volunteer clergy which can create an inter-disciplinary void. There may be a high percentage of patients who do not have a church affinity but request culturally sensitive and faith-system-sensitive spiritual care in times of crisis, they deserve nothing less. There are training manuals available that provide good information for Auxiliary Directors and Volunteer Coordinators as they seek to   equip area clergy who have had no formal Clinical Pastoral Education training. And once again, never assume that area clergy have received formal training in college, seminary or in their ordination process that would equip them for all the things they will encounter in the clinical environment. The Association of Clinical Pastoral Education and the College of Pastoral Supervision and Psychotherapy have projected Standards of Practice for Professional Chaplains (9) which should, at a minimum, provide the standards for any model of Pastoral Care delivery.

Here is another if which comes to mind. If the Auxiliary Director or Volunteer Coordinator is entrusted with the responsibility to contact the patient's clergy or church for spiritual care, what happens if that patient's clergyperson is not available or in cases where the church is without a pastor? What should be done when a patient does not want his or her clergyperson notified under any circumstances, for fear that his or her name will appear in the church bulletin or on a prayer list without their permission? (Such an event in the healthcare setting would be a violation of federal privacy requirements spelled out in the HIPAA law, which could result in fines, penalties and, possibly, litigation). What if your patient's pastor cannot follow up in short order? Sometimes it can take a while for them to be notified and even longer before they arrive. Let's face it, when a clergy person is present, the patient's needs may or may not be met. It is our hope their clergy person will do an effective job so that the patient will be more at ease with their circumstances and ultimately able to connect up with their plan of care.

Director of Pastoral Care utilizing contract Chaplains
In order to maintain Joint Commission accreditation and not totally eliminate Pastoral Care services, many hospitals have a Director of Pastoral Care on staff, who utilizes contract Chaplains as a cost-saving measure and still provide 24/7 coverage. The contract Chaplains may be CPE trained or be trained by the Director of Pastoral Care as to the organization's priority of needs. There are a few free standing pastoral care entities (such as Lutheran Chaplain Services in Cleveland, Ohio (10)), who contract with Directors of Pastoral Care and/or Administrators to provide Chaplain services for a fee. Contract Chaplains are recruited by the free standing entity to provide Pastoral Care and Presence as needed. In most cases, at the end of the year the contract Chaplain will receive a 1099 form for tax purposes. Like volunteer clergy, contract Chaplains are less likely to become integrated as a member of the inter-disciplinary

team. They normally focus on patient and family Pastoral Care needs when paged and not so much on the needs of the medical staff. A Contract Chaplains' level of attachment to the hospital and integration with the staff can closely parallel that of registry nurses, who work intermittently or contract on for brief stints and then move to the next hospital in need of their service. There may be times when the Director of Pastoral Care will use contract Chaplains if budget constraints warrant. Utilizing contract Chaplain's requires careful scheduling and a good backup plan in case someone calls to say they cannot respond for one reason or another. Who will cover then? Contract Chaplains are used more commonly for nights and weekends and they are paid a fee for being on call and then an hourly wage when they respond in person to a death or trauma.

PRN Chaplains (as needed)

Another trend in Pastoral Care within the corporate setting includes the utilization of PRN (as needed) Chaplains instead of paying full-time wages. Normally they are utilized during high census times and whenever the budget allows. The Director will contact PRN Chaplains when they determine that a need exists for their services. These Chaplains are paid an hourly fee and some of them are likely to be those who at one time held a full time position in the Pastoral Care department. They know that they are present (as needed) to address the Pastoral Care needs within the clinical setting. The important issue for Administration to consider is if Pastoral Care is readily available at times when special needs arise. What about the times when mass casualty events occur in your community and your PRN people are not available? While the PRN option may seem to be a sufficient means of staffing in some hospitals, it is often merely a means to reduce labor costs. Once again, this model may fall short in meeting the personal needs of nurses, physicians or ancillary staff who may want to process. If a Director of Pastoral Care is the only staff person and PRN staff is utilized, it places a large responsibility upon the Director to keep up during low census times. The acuity level during low census at times may be higher than during high census times. Pastoral Care, particularly in times of crisis, is time-sensitive. Studies have shown that it is important to be present as quickly as possible during the impact stage of grief. Chaplains need as much "heads up" time as possible when events occur.

Using Chaplains on a PRN basis clearly is a cost-conscious strategy, designed to meet basic Pastoral Care needs of patients and their families while keeping the department budget in focus. The following is an example of a "help wanted" ad a hospital might place in a newspaper or on-line job-posting site, seeking applicants for a PRN Chaplain position.

Pastoral Care - Chaplain
Per Diem

Hours:	As needed – Days, weekends, Overnight on-call/weekends
Job Details:	**Basic Functions:** To respond to emergency "codes" and patient deaths that occur during the day, evening/night shift, weekends and

on other occasions when needed.

Requirements:

1. B.A./B.S. degree preferred. Associate's degree (or equivalent amount of college credits) in psychosocial, theological or related field required.
2. A minimum of three years' experience in Pastoral Care preferred.
3. One unit of CPE or equivalent experience, such as pastor (in good standing) of a church in a recognized denomination.

Nursing staff and Case Managers meeting spiritual needs

While there always will be nursing staff (and others) in the hospital setting who are deeply religious and/or spiritual and more than willing to "hone in" on a patient's perceived need. Intentionally utilizing or allowing them to address a patient's religious, spiritual and sacramental needs is another trend. Not only does it not meet Joint Commission standards for a spiritual assessment by a qualified person, it sets up the hospital for significant challenges. Recently, there was a nurse whose husband was on staff at a large church in our community. She worked in surgery and would intentionally do pre-op visits with patients going in for surgery and those patients who were in our ICU. Her visit would include telling them her name, what church she attended and something about their programs at her church that she thought might interest them or fit the situation. She promoted her church and its programs quite well. Rarely did she leave the visit without trying to link that person up with someone she thought would follow up with them. That particular church also had a staff member, a former healthcare worker himself, whose specific focus was ministry to healthcare professionals. He would solicit healthcare workers to be a Christian witness to patients and to lead them to salvation, if the opportunity presented itself. While one can appreciate the religious zeal exhibited by devout employees who work in healthcare, it is imperative that one remember that the patient is there for healthcare reasons and should not be unduly subjected to evangelism or proselytism. Such practices can create role confusion and subvert good Pastoral Care services. Most nurses have not received the formal theological or clinical pastoral training required to conduct an accurate spiritual assessment, and their religious or spiritual enthusiasm alone is not sufficient to address the myriad of Pastoral Care challenges and needs that exist inside the walls of a hospital.

Those administrators who advocate a particular religious viewpoint may allow or even encourage nurses and other staff members to address the spiritual needs of patients as they arise. While this mindset reflects a perspective of patient care that may be well-intended, it can quickly become a distraction from professional care for the whole person. Administrators who allow too much dabbling in spiritual areas by nursing staff need to be more aware of how quality pastoral care and presence impacts HCAHPS, the community, patient needs and the bottom line.

Another developing trend in corporate healthcare is to incorporate spiritual care and family systems needs into the role of a nurse Case Manager. Many for-profit hospitals and health systems have replaced Social Workers with Case Managers. The Case Manager's primary role is to oversee the patient's hospital stay and transition to home or another healthcare setting and coordinate with health plans on coverage and reimbursement issues. A Case Manager's job description usually prescribes that they help develop a plan of care, monitor patient progress, assess patient care, ensure the quality of care is high and determine what best suits the patient's needs. They are patient advocates, as well as agents working toward the most efficient, cost-conscious care on behalf of the insurance provider and the medical facility, but they are not professional Pastoral Care providers.

The inter-disciplinary team focus slips farther away when this model is in place. Just as a significant difference exists between a nurse Case Manager who has no social work experience and a Licensed Certified Social Worker who has specialized training, even a larger skill-set difference exists between a nurse Case Manager and a clinically trained Pastoral Care provider. In most hospitals that utilize this model, nurse Case Managers, are required to address a patient's needs from the time they hit the door until the time they are discharged. This often includes addressing the psychosocial-spiritual needs of the patient. The corporate rationale seems to be, since Case Managers work closely with the patient from admission to discharge on the aforementioned issues, why not utilize them to address spiritual issues in patients as they arise. While it may be possible to train a nurse Case Manager to function on such a multi-faceted professional level, keeping up with the sheer volume of work on such a broad professional spectrum would be a daunting task. The most concerning aspect of this trend for me is the loss of inter-disciplinary functioning within the healthcare environment. This approach is relegated to a reliance on a nurse to do everything and is doomed to fall short of meeting the patients' needs in the spiritual and religious domain.

One of our CFOs once asked if I could have a social worker cover for me when I was asked to "flex" (take vacation or unpaid leave) during periods of low patient census. Of course I told him his idea would not work at all, since there is quite a difference in our roles. His question told me that he did not realize that we no longer had Social Workers in our health system; they had been replaced by nurse Case Managers. It became an opportunity for me to educate him on the role of a Pastoral Care professional and how we differed from a Nurse Case Manager.

Director of Culture and Diversity overseeing Pastoral Care services

William Mott (11) said, the world is getting smaller, in terms of cultural integration. Healthcare centers are hiring Directors of Culture and Diversity who are working alongside Directors of Pastoral Care and, in some cases, are in charge of putting together a Pastoral Care team. In many hospice organizations, social workers serve as bereavement coordinators who not only take on culture and diversity issues but also coordinate Pastoral Care services for people in hospice care.

In large cities and small town America a growing mix of cultures are represented. It is my belief that the composition of hospital staff in general and Pastoral Care staff in particular should mirror the community it serves. Embracing cultural customs and beliefs of a diverse patient and community population is an integral part of respecting the patient and delivering quality care. We want to treat them the way they want to be treated. The practice of monitoring the effectiveness of culture and diversity programs within a hospital or healthcare system is an ongoing process. Hospitals and healthcare systems must be committed to equity and fairness in staff and patient care. In some hospitals, Pastoral Care is directly involved in culture and diversity sensitivity training, while in others the trend is to make it a responsibility of the Director of Culture and Diversity.

When I walk into a patient's room, culture and diversity assessment is as natural as introducing myself, as it should be for Pastoral Care providers, nursing staff and all who have patient contact. Cultural differences that a patient expects to be honored should be clearly and appropriately communicated by them at the point of admission. In many hospitals, cultural issues and/or requests are clearly addressed in admission and patient rights forms that are filled out when the patient is admitted. Culturally sensitive healthcare is considered a human right, and the Joint Commission spells out that expectation in the RI standards that were mentioned previously.

Directors of Pastoral Care in multiple leadership roles

We all know that consolidating as many services as possible, to save on labor costs, is a commonly employed practice in healthcare these days. It is not uncommon for a Director of Pastoral Care to manage additional departments and chair several committees, some of which I have already mentioned. Reviewing resumes for Director of Pastoral Care positions will shed some light on this trend. However, I caution Directors of Pastoral Care about wearing too many hats in their hospital or healthcare system because it can become counter-productive and present inappropriate inter-connectedness. While diversification in your financial portfolio may work well, it does not benefit a Director of Pastoral Care to "wear too many hats" in a healthcare setting. When the Chair of the Institutional Review Board is also the Chair of the Biomedical Ethics Committee and an audit of both panels occurs, it is an invitation for an undue, and perhaps unwanted, level of scrutiny. Also, any high-performing professional can experience a decrease in effectiveness if he or she is "spread too thin" by taking on too many areas of responsibility. Overload is a stress inducer, and good staff can experience true "burnout" when expected to do too much. When employees are over worked, their productivity levels can drop, creativity may be stymied and morale deeply affected. Vocational overload is directly linked to increased anxiety, fatigue, depression, physiological stress and an erosion of one's sense of purpose. Not only are the effects felt personally, families may very well feel them, too.

Palliative Care and Pastoral Care Services

While palliative care programs have been up and going in many hospitals for some time, the continuing rapid growth in hospice services has challenged hospitals to get on board. Palliative care medicine is a focus on enhancing quality of life for patients and family members facing life-limiting conditions. Palliative measures focus on advance care planning, complex symptom management, psychosocial and spiritual support, assistance with end-of-life decisions, continuity of care, bereavement services and inter-disciplinary teamwork throughout the process. To relieve suffering, healthcare must bring inter-disciplinary expertise together to treat the whole person. Due to the growing need for Chaplains in hospice organizations in our community, the CPE program that I supervise offers a specific palliative care and hospice specialty focus. More and more nurses and physicians are acquiring accreditation in this area. There is also a growing interest in Thanatology within our society with those in fields such as nursing, psychology, psychiatry, religious studies, sociology and social work becoming certified. Thanatology is the academic and scientific study of death.

Referring patients to Behavioral Health professionals for grief issues

While this is happening more often, it may not rise to the level of a trend. We know that Pastoral Care services are not billable; these services are provided by the hospital for its patients, family members and staff. If a hospital has a behavioral health unit that is staffed with a psychologist, psychiatrist, APNs (advance practice nurses) and others whose services are billable, there's a good chance patients are being referred to them to address grief issues and other symptoms that Chaplains in the past have addressed.

The optimum for any hospital or healthcare system is to experience consistent bottom line and top line growth. While some areas are losing population density, our healthcare system is in an area of the country that is experiencing rapid growth, even during our recent time of economic recession. (12) In the middle of the recession, when we were experiencing staff reductions, it was easy to site recession factors as the cause. However, during times of rapid population growth and expansion when the economy has rebounded, the corporate expectation still seems to be to add new service lines without adding staff. And, again, that practice leads to overload and staff "burnout."

REVIEWING: What do you see emerging from these trends? What has been occurring in your hospital or healthcare system that you need to make note of as a director?

Chapter Three- Pastoral Presence

While a whirlwind of changes and challenges are on the horizon for healthcare reform in America, some basic needs in the soul of humanity always will be present, no matter what the face of healthcare looks like in the future. Humans will continue to confront trauma, loss, end-of-life issues, loneliness, weakness, vulnerabilities, fallen spirits and medical, religious and spiritual dilemmas. These maladies will never end, as long as humanity exists. As Lewis B. Smedes wrote in his book, "A Pretty Good Person," (13) "the strongest and brightest of us are fragile as a floating bubble, unsteady as a newborn kitten on a waxed kitchen floor." One minute, life is rocking on in peace and tranquility, and the next minute, a crisis can take it all away. Healthcare always will benefit from Pastoral Care professionals who are appropriately compassionate, skilled at empowering patients, effective patient advocates, engaged inter-disciplinary team members, culture-builders and are also ready and committed to graciously enter difficult conversations, when needed.

Pastoral presence is not about curing a disease or taking away the patient's pain as much as it is providing a caring and healing demeanor and walking with him or her as the pain leads to a new reality. Carol Taylor, in the Supportive Voice (Vol. 11, No. 2; summer 2006), wrote, (14) "curing is the alleviation of symptoms or the termination of suppression of a disease process through surgical, chemical, or mechanical intervention. Healing may be spontaneous, but more often it's a gradual awakening to a deeper sense of self (and of the self in relation to others) in a way that effects profound change. Healing comes from within and is consistent with a person's own readiness to grow and to change. A healing attitude is a belief system that recognizes that all of life's experiences, including injury, illness and other setbacks, provide us with opportunities to learn and to grow toward that which we are meant to be. Seen in this light, disease is not an enemy but a teacher and motivation. Disease is manifesting, in a physical way, the desire or need of the psyche to re-establish balance and integration, through a change of direction in one's lifestyle, behavior, or attitudes." This is the exact dimension where medical science and Pastoral Care blend like coffee and cream.

While providing pastoral presence, one does not project his or her beliefs on the patient. As America becomes more acculturated, spirituality is becoming more accepted than denominational loyalty. Pastoral Care providers must be able to function within that milieu. A Pastoral Care provider who is versed in world religions and age-specific spiritual dimensions will find paths that are easier to navigate. Leaving personal agenda aside and going where the patient needs to go is essential. Clinical Pastoral Education taught in a clinical environment exposes students to a multitude of crisis and trauma situations. The student is afforded the opportunity to reflect theologically, spiritually, emotionally and relationally in that environment. It is a combination of cognitive and affective learning opportunities that allows them to get in touch with the Self in a dynamic way. (Note: "Self" is the term I will use hereafter to refer to a person's spiritual core, the embodiment of who he or she is and what he or she believes. I capitalize Self as a proper noun because I believe it to be a person, as opposed to the different personas we exhibit in changing circumstances. Self is who we truly are, not just who we merely project ourselves to be or the face we "put on" for a certain occasion or situation.) Unless Pastoral Care providers are extremely secure with their own internal, spiritual identities, they will be prone to getting caught up in their own issues, while trying to be present for others. Often, I tell Pastoral Care interns that it is difficult for a Pastoral Care provider to be present for people who are in great emotional pain if his or her own unresolved pain is triggered in the process. Emotional, theological, spiritual and relational issues that a Pastoral Care provider has not processed will be triggered at some time during a visit, and this usually takes place when he or she least expects it.

The hospital is a microcosm of the community, where Pastoral Care providers meet all types of people, in all types of circumstances. Trauma and every family dynamic under the sun can be found in a healthcare setting at one time or another. A Pastoral Care provider is exposed to the core of human nature, even as they work on their knowledge of Self and attempt to be present for people in pain.

COMPASSION

In healthcare today, there appears to be a constant struggle to keep compassionate care at the forefront for patients. There probably are many factors involved in this dynamic, but unless a person is drawn to healthcare out of some compassion for people in pain, learning to be compassionate may be quite a journey. While some healthcare workers have the innate ability to be compassionate toward patients during difficult times in life, extending true compassion to hurting people is not easy for most healthcare workers. As a result, an attempt at compassion often comes out as empty platitudes. Unresolved issues in the lives of people who are attempting to minister to people in crisis often get triggered, and the would-be comforters find themselves wrapped up on their own blankets of need. Even people who are professionally trained in providing Pastoral Care and presence may struggle with providing appropriate compassion to those who most need it. In my experience with training interns to become Pastoral Care providers, I have noticed that even students who otherwise are quite proficient at practicing the skills required to provide Pastoral Care may struggle at mastering the element of compassion.

Two root words that I see in "compassion" help me gain a deeper perspective on how to appropriately and effectively extend it. The first word is "compass." A compass is an instrument for determining direction, often when direction is needed most. People who need compassion often have lost their sense of direction and need "True North" to steady them, as they search for new direction or a new reality. Let's face it, events in life can spin us so fast that when we are left to stand on our own, we are dizzy and struggle to know which way to go and how to steady ourselves in a wobbly attempt to walk again. A compassionate caregiver who knows Self in a dynamic way can, in the midst of a crisis, can become "True North" for that wandering soul. Giving of themselves on a regular basis, compassionate caregivers must ask themselves, "Where is this leading me?" After providing compassion to people in deep crisis, one must decompress by taking pause and setting aside time for a period of reflection and "centering."

The second word I see in the word "compassion" is "passion," which is defined, in part, as a powerful or compelling emotion or feeling that often moves us to action. Pastoral Care providers who become entangled in the emotional experiences of the people they are serving must take their "emotional pulse," as well. Following are some questions that Pastoral Care providers should ask themselves in such situations:

- "What emotions are driving me to help this person or family?"
- "How healthy and helpful are those emotions?"
- "When have I experienced similar emotions?

- Do I need to revisit a past experience to experience
  further growth?"
- "What do I need to do in the present to keep my
  emotions in check?"

If a Pastoral Care provider fails to do his or her inner work, compassion fatigue lurks just around the corner.

In the search to understand the essence of compassion, Henri J.M. Nouwen said, (15) "Let us not underestimate how hard it is to be compassionate. Compassion is hard because it requires the inner disposition to go with others to places where they are weak, vulnerable, lonely, and broken. What we desire most is to do away with suffering by fleeing from it or finding a quick cure for it." In providing pastoral presence, we must be clear about our sense of passion and where it may lead us. Is the Pastoral Care professional willing and able to go where his or her passion may dictate?

EMPOWERING THE PATIENT

A Pastoral Care provider's focus is to be present for those who are in crisis. Being present does not mean taking away emotional pain but going where the people need to go and empowering them to tell their own stories.

While blood panels may help tell a physician what is going on with a patient in a chemical and/or systemic sense, there may be feelings, churning in the pit of a person's stomach, that are having as much of an effect on that person as a virus or bacterium. Offering the person an opportunity to name that feeling and explore what is behind it is priceless for many. "What's going on?" is a question that can open the door for a meaningful journey inward.

Just spend a few moments thinking about how much personal information people are required to give as they access healthcare. Once the registration technician has extracted all the facts he or she needs to adequately establish a patient's identity, insurance coverage, ability to pay for services (which includes recent credit history), etc., then he or she enters into the consent-for-treatment phase, followed by all those questions involving HIPAA and protected health information. "Sign here and initial here and here in the highlighted spaces," the registration technician says. Once the patient has been through registration, he or she meets with a Triage Nurse, who asks for more information about pain, symptoms and past medical history. Answers to these questions can provide clues as to what should be done to address the patient's needs. The patient's condition, relative to other patients seeking healthcare, will be evaluated and ranked to establish diagnostic and treatment priorities.

Once the patient finally sees a healthcare provider, giving more information about himself or herself starts again. After the provider's initial assessment, he or she often will order tests, to gather even more information. "We need to take a urine sample, do some lab work, do an ultrasound or CT, monitor your vital signs, etc.," the patient may hear a healthcare provider say. Then a nurse may tell the patient that he or she needs a certain medicine or even give instructions not to eat or drink for a certain period of time prior to another test or procedure. And, of course, nothing is immediate – the patient frequently has to anxiously wait (perhaps hours or even days) to learn the results of tests.

While many culture-building programs stress keeping the patient informed, the bottom line is that the patient has entered a process of information-giving that they hope will lead to an understanding of what is going on inside his or her body and result in a diagnosis. Once a patient has received a diagnosis, the demand for information decreases as the medical team takes over with a treatment plan. However, in the patient's mind, there is more to tell – the story goes on. But who will listen? A Pastoral Care provider knows how to listen for themes, words and phrases that are used in a patient's story and clarify them for a more complete understanding of what is going on in the patient's life. This process leads to a more complete picture of the patient's emotional and spiritual condition.

In Quint Studer's book, "Hardwiring Excellence," he advocates AIDET, an acronym for Acknowledge-Introduce-Duration-Explanation-Thank You. (16) These steps have proven to help reduce anxiety in patients and improve patient-satisfaction scores. AIDET is a simple method of prompting healthcare workers to be personable and let patients know who they are, what they are there to do and how long the activity will take. While this is scripting to a degree, it is at least an attempt to help nursing staff and others who enter the patient's world to be informative. When providing pastoral presence, the Pastoral Care provider goes much farther and empowers the patient. Pastoral presence helps a patient explore the emotional and spiritual dimensions of life, so he or she can engage more completely with his or her plan of care and the "new normal" that they will be experiencing after hospitalization.

CNN Senior Medical Correspondent Elizabeth Cohen wanted to be an empowered patient because of her infant daughter's experience in a Neonatal Intensive Care Unit, so she started a column on CNN's website, addressing the concept of empowerment of patients. In her research, she discovered that about 99,000 people die each year from infections they acquire in hospitals. She also states that diagnoses will be wrong as many as 1-in-4 times. She has written a book, "The Empowered Patient," (17) which is based on her research.

An article in the December 2003 edition of the Joint Commission Journal on Quality and Safety ("Patient Centeredness – Addressing Patients' Emotional and Spiritual Needs") (18) reported that an analysis of Press-Ganey Associates' 2001 National Inpatient Database showed a strong link between the mission of Pastoral Care and patient satisfaction. The article stated that survey data collected from 1,732,562 patients between January 2001 and December 2001 revealed a strong relationship between the "degree to which staff addressed emotional/spiritual needs" and overall patient satisfaction. Three measurements most highly correlated with emotional/spiritual care were:

- Staff response to concerns/complaints.
- Staff efforts to include patients in decisions about treatment.
- Staff sensitivity to the inconvenience that health problems and hospitalization can cause.

The concept of empowering the patient is not a new one. Back when physicians made house calls, they would spend time listening to the patient, observing the home environment and "taking it all in" as a part of the process of diagnosing and treating their patients. There is much to be gleaned from patients, and those in healthcare who empower patients to tell their own stories and come away with a deeper understanding of what is truly going on. That which is learned from a patient's story is used to construct a more complete treatment plan that may result in greater success. Who knows better about what's going on than the patient? In today's healthcare, we need to revive a greater interest in the patient's life and story as we seek to provide compassionate care and healing.

Empowerment, from a Pastoral Care perspective, begins the moment a Chaplain or Pastoral Care provider enters the patient's room. Patients should expect nothing less than to be empowered. A Pastoral Care provider's objective is to go where patients need to go during the visit. Pastoral Care providers must leave their agendas outside the door, realizing that the process is not about them – it's truly all about the patient. A Pastoral Care provider who has processed his or her life thoroughly and dynamically will have little problem with personal issues being triggered. In cases in which a Pastoral Care provider is experiencing "fresh" pain or grief and becomes too close to a situation, he or she must recognize that fact and back away, allowing someone else to take over.

Staff empowerment of patients is a vital sign of a healthy hospital or healthcare system. Words or phrases such as,

"Tell me what's going on" and/or, "What feelings are churning inside?" empowers patients to go where they need to go. These types of questions can quickly move the conversation and care to a deeper level. So how does a Pastoral Care provider go about empowering the patient and staying away from his or her own personal agenda, religious dogma or anything else that might pollute the process? Let's look at the following exchange between a patient, spouse, children and the Pastoral Care provider or Chaplain.

Chaplain: "Hello, my name is Chaplain C.J. … Your name is … ? (keeping good eye contact with the patient, to prevent others in the room from diverting focus from the patient).

Patient: "My name is William, but I go by Bill."

Chaplain: (Still focused on the patient) "I see you have some other folks here with you. How are they connected to you?" (This empowers Bill to make those introductions. It is important to stay focused on the patient, even as others in the room try to interject and introduce themselves. They get the hint that the Chaplain is focusing in on Bill and begin to respect the conversation.)

Patient: "This is Jane, and she's my wife. This is Chris, and he's my son. This is B.J.; she's my daughter, and Tim, her husband."

Chaplain: (Briefly acknowledging them and immediately turning back to the patient) "Looks like you have a lot of family support here with you. Would you like for me to come back later?"

Patient: "No. They don't mind. We're all family."

Patient's son: "Dad, I'm going to go down to the cafeteria for a few minutes. (At this announcement, the rest of the family – except for the patient's wife – thinks that is a good idea and excuse themselves, as well.)

Patient's wife: (Immediately after the rest of the family exits, she seizes an opportunity to talk. As the Chaplain stays focused on the patient, his wife begins to speak.) "Chaplain, Bill is so positive about things, but the doctor is not. Could you talk to him about how he really feels about what is going on? It doesn't look good, and I know it has to be bothering him. We just want him to know how much we love him and need him."

Chaplain: (Still focused on the patient and noticing that the patient rolled his eyes ever so slightly as his wife was talking.) "Bill, how are things?

Patient: "I'm O.K with things."

Chaplain: "O.K. with things?"

Patient: "Yes. I know I'm in bad shape, but I'm O.K. with it."

Chaplain: "Bad shape?" (Then pausing, waiting for him to clarify that statement.)

Patient: "I'm going to die, Chaplain. But I've lived a good life, and I have a lovely family. They are the light of my life, and I certainly will miss them, but we don't live forever, you know."

Chaplain: (Pausing to assess the moment, the Chaplain hears the sound of the patient's wife gently sobbing as she stands at the foot of the bed and then see an immediate shift in the patient's demeanor. The patient's "tough-man" facade begins to crack. As the patient glances at his wife, his eyes wet with tears. This couple needs time alone.) "I see some tears. Sounds like you two have connected. Where do you need to go from here?"

Patient and wife: (No words necessary. The patient's wife moves to the side of the bed and leans over to kiss her husband. They embrace. They have been empowered, and they both are capable of doing their own work from this point forward. Empowering them in this context provides a breath of fresh air, relieving built-up tension. The children had sensed it too and were hoping for some resolution. Empowering the patient to do or say what he or she needs to say or do is a powerful dynamic. The rest of the conversation was open and filled with a new sense of acceptance.)

Many physicians struggle with knowing how to empower patients and stay focused on them in the midst of a visit in which several family members are present. During a visit where I was present with one of our Pulmonologists, this very thing happened. After the visit, we spent some time reflecting on it, and he asked me how I handle those situations in which the presence of family members makes communication with the patient a real challenge. That question was an opportunity for me to share with him the concept of empowerment and how to stay focused on the patient, almost to the exclusion of the family, when necessary. This keeps a clear path open and lets others present know the subject of my visit. As a Chaplain, I learn a lot about the patient's family dynamics during my visits. The main objective is to enable the patient to hear his or her own voice. Voice equals choice! If the patient's voice is heard, then he or she is more apt to make informed choices and take an active role in his or her plan of care and treatment options.

DIFFICULT CONVERSATIONS

Having those difficult conversations is often what patients, family members, staff and physicians fear the most. While they know what needs to be conveyed, gaining the courage to convey it overwhelms them. Not being intimidated by entering difficult conversations is important, since many patients can pick up easily on what others are projecting. Be confident that the message that needs to be conveyed will be delivered and that a good outcome ultimately will be experienced by all involved.

When my father was weaned from the ventilator, after yet another episode of intubation, due to congestive heart failure (CHF) and chronic obstructive pulmonary disease (COPD), I spoke with the Pulmonologist to gain his perspective. He told me that this would be an on-going pattern for Dad from here on out. After extubation, my father asked me what had happened. I said, "Dad, the doctor said your lungs are bad, and they keep filling up with fluid, which causes you to experience difficulty in breathing, and the level of oxygen saturation in your blood drops off. When that happens, they have to intubate you to get your saturation levels up again. He turned to me and spoke in a clear and resolved voice, saying, "I've had enough. No more!" Of course, I knew what that meant, but my mother and seven other siblings needed to hear it, too. A few minutes later, my Dad summoned us all into the room and told us that the end was near for him and that he wanted no more of this. As a large sibling group, we had just witnessed our father's verbal advance directive, but we needed to go through our own process of accepting it, knowing full well what that entailed – the death of our father. We all sat in a room and cast our vote to honor his wishes, with our eldest brother objecting. He and my father had been like brothers for more than 58 years and had seen many fun times and challenges together. He simply wasn't ready to let him go, and we all understood how deeply this was impacting him. He was not only losing a father, he was losing his closest friend. We honored my father's wishes, and he died peacefully at home, with hospice care.

A short five years later, our mother was facing a difficult diagnosis and prognosis. She had a sore on her foot that became infected and led to sepsis (a systemic infection) and sick serum syndrome, a rare blood disorder. During this process, her fever would rise, but as the high-powered antibiotics did their work, it would decrease. Up and down it went. She was decrepit and could barely walk before this development, and now, her knees seemed to be frozen. She did not have the energy or the willpower to move at all. Being bedridden was the best we could hope for, and somehow she knew it. We had one of those difficult conversations with her, explaining what we knew and allowing her to do her processing. She had told us over the years that she never wanted to be a burden to anyone, and she knew that she would be from that day forward. Once again, we siblings gathered together to discuss Mom and process her wishes. This was another difficult conversation for all of us, but we knew it needed to happen. Two weeks later, she died peacefully at home, with hospice care.

Once difficult conversations are entered into, they can be very cathartic for everyone involved. However, avoiding them will only lead to more "stuffed" feelings and elevated levels of anxiety. Addressing a difficult conversation with a patient who is dying or telling an employee he or she is not meeting expectations and/or that his or her employment is being terminated is best done directly, honestly and compassionately. During their clinical training, Pastoral Care providers have many opportunities to enter difficult conversations with patients, family, staff and physicians. They also enter difficult conversations with their peer groups on a regular basis. It is in these sessions that they learn to confront, clarify and give and receive feedback, which gets them started toward handling difficult conversations in other settings.

Pastoral Care providers know that processing difficult conversations with patients and family members often begins with empowering them to go where they need to go. Tracking with patients often takes a Pastoral Care provider to the core of their issues. What I often have discovered is that patients already have processed issues with which others are still struggling. Difficult conversations can be a real challenge for physicians, nursing staff and for mid-level managers and administrators. How does the person initiating a difficult dialogue go about saying what needs to be said? First of all, be certain that the information being communicated is accurate. It is not ethical to heighten a person's anxiety over something that is not a fact or certainty. I have heard many stories from patients and family members who have been told that a test or exam has detected something that likely may be cancerous, but a ruling from Pathology is needed to positively identify the problem. Obviously, the patient's and family's anxiety is heightened. This anxiety is only compounded by having to wait for an undetermined amount of time for the final results. Secondly, communicate the facts directly. (Example: "Mrs. Smith, I'm Chaplain C.J., and I heard the doctor say that the CT scan revealed that you have a dissecting aortic aneurism that is not repairable. Mrs. Smith, this is sure to result in your death." In this example, the Pastoral Care provider should allow time for the patient to process this information, and if she is alert and oriented enough, she may have something to say to the Chaplain or her family. The Chaplain's role is to be present and helpful, so that any communication the patient wants to accomplish can happen sooner, rather than later. Thirdly, be honest with the patient as he or she poses questions. Finally, be compassionate and present for the patient. The Chaplain may be the last person to visit with him or her in this temporal setting.

BEING PASTORAL

How is it possible that someone can enter a room filled with anxious people and become a non-anxious presence bringing calm to them? How are Pastoral Care providers able to go to those dark places of the soul where patients are trapped and provide the opportunity for them to find their way out?

One weekday morning in the fall of 2009 (around 10:30 a.m.) an EMS page came into the Emergency Department. An 8-year-old student from a local elementary school had collapsed on the playground. As with any Pediatric emergency, staff experienced a heightened sense of anxiety. Many of the nurses working that morning had children of a similar age. They had sent their own kids off to school earlier. As you might imagine, many things were going through their minds as they searched for additional information about this elementary student. "What school did you say the student was attending?" "What was the age again?" As we later learned from the child's mother, the little girl had not complained of any severe pain or discomfort prior to her collapse. At most, she had displayed symptoms similar to a slight cold and runny nose, not accompanied by fever, congestion or other symptoms out of the ordinary. She loved school and would not want to miss for any reason. Her teacher and others supervising the playground said she was running and playing with her classmates just before she collapsed. The school nurse, EMS personnel and medical staff worked feverishly to save her life, but her heart had stopped. After attempting resuscitation for 40 minutes in the Emergency Department, the Code Blue was called off, and she was pronounced dead. Her body was sent to the state Medical Examiner's office. Later, we learned she had a congenital heart anomaly. I might add that when those types of deaths occur or when small children are air-lifted to a larger children's hospital, staff do not have closure unless the receiving hospital provides an update. Pastoral Care providers in our system decompress with staff in Pediatric trauma cases, so that they do not take the stress of the event home to their families. I was present with the mother and father during that most difficult time, listening to their words of sorrow and love being poured out over their beautiful daughter. They experienced the impact stage of grief and moments of disbelief as they finally spoke words that demonstrated some measure of acceptance: "She looks so peaceful ... like an angel lying there. But I don't want to let her go!"

Those experiencing deep anxiety or who are in the impact stage of grief benefit from someone being present with them who has the ability to simply be there without interjecting empty platitudes or a personal agenda. A Pastoral Care provider who has specialized training in the art of Pastoral Care and who is deeply relational is able to do that very thing. Being present for people in great emotional pain is possible when Pastoral Care professionals have processed their own pain to the extent that it is not triggered by the circumstances and experiences of others. This doesn't mean that things don't bother them. Being human means that there will be events experienced in life and in the healthcare setting that will tug at our heart strings. It means Pastoral Care providers have learned to balance the cognitive and affective domains and realize that the hurting people are experiencing deep emotional pain and need a special someone to be present in those moments.

There are times when a Pastoral Care provider will walk away from a visit in deep theological reflection over what he or she has just experienced and realizing that the visit was exactly what was needed for him or her to grow spiritually or theologically.

FAMILY SYSTEMS

As I work with families in the hospital who are in the midst of a physical crisis or impending death, I remind myself that they are tangled balls of emotions, searching for a way to unscramble what they are experiencing. As a Pastoral Care provider, I am there to "mid-wife" that experience.

When paged to the Emergency Department for a trauma situation, entering the consultation room where family members have gathered is a critical first step. Before I enter the room, I make sure that I have as much information as possible about what is going on. That means talking with the ED physician, nurse, department supervisor, House Supervisor or whomever I can to get factual information – I want to be informed! As I open the door, I say, "Hello, I'm Chaplain C.J. I don't want to alarm you unnecessarily, but our hospital pages the Chaplain when we have a trauma or Code Blue in our ED." Introducing oneself as a Chaplain can create a reaction from a family member that may need to be addressed at some time, so I keep a close eye on reactions when I introduce myself. Being observant at this moment also helps me gain insight into the family's "emotional skin."

In order to understand the family system better, I ask how everyone is connected to the patient. To get a handle on how large a family this might be, I ask if there are others on their way or if there are others they will be contacting. If other family members already are on their way, I ask how long it might take for them to arrive. Answers to these questions help me identify the possible spokesperson, who also may be the decision-maker as we continue to walk with them through this event. Next, I ask them to tell me what has happened. It is important for them to tell their stories of what transpired and to connect all the events in their minds. It is especially helpful as they seek to find their way through a snarled web of emotions and connect up to a new reality. By this point, I have established my role and set the family more at ease, so that they can concentrate their energies on processing what is happening. Often, I see loved ones struggle to dial numbers on their cell phones, search frantically for a piece of paper or retrieve an item from a purse. It is important to remain calm and allow them to work through their struggles, since this process really does help them make sense of what they are experiencing.

For some patients and/or family members, the title of Chaplain will have a negative connotation or one that they equate with a pastor and perhaps an adverse church experience. Be patient when that becomes apparent. Some people exhibit anger in the impact stage of grief and unleash some pretty specific vernacular to state how they feel about clergy and preachers. Additionally, I have encountered people who did not even want me to be around them because, in their minds, the presence of a Chaplain portended a possible death and meant they would have to give up hoping for a positive outcome. Why else would a Chaplain be present? "If it is bad enough to call the Chaplain, it must be really bad" is the line of thinking.

A Chaplain steeped in the art of Pastoral Care will be an inter-disciplinary team member who possesses the ability to assess a crisis situation and provide the care and calming presence needed in the moment. A Chaplain who has learned the art of Pastoral Care well will be able to integrate several theories into a comprehensive assessment of what he or she is experiencing. A Chaplain has learned to practice a unique set of skills to positively impact people who are suffering.

PATIENT ADVOCATE

The Chaplain serves as a patient advocate in matters that may keep patients from participating in their plans of care. If those issues are not resolved by an objective person, they will fester and be reflected in patient-satisfaction scores. When I am paged by a nurse to visit a patient who is being difficult, one of the first questions that I ask the nurse is, "What's going on?" As I am listening to him or her explain how difficult the patient has been, I also observe the nurse and will ask, "How are things with you?" or "How are you handling all this?" It is amazing how often I find that the tolerance level of the nurse has been affected by a personal or work issue, and all it took was a difficult patient to tip the scales. Once I have assessed the nurse, I also assess the patient by empowering him or her to tell his or her story. It never ceases to amaze me how things outside the scope of a patient's pain level, diagnosis and prognosis can factor into their behavior. On one particular occasion, I was paged to the room of a patient who the nurse described as being very agitated. Upon entering the room and empowering the patient, I asked the question, "How are things?" The patient's immediate response was, "Not so good." "Not so good?" I asked. "Tell me more about that." The patient then took the opportunity to share with me that he did not have health insurance and that with each test he was told would be needed, he became angrier, since he did not know how he would be able to pay his bill. Another patient, who was dying, was concerned about who would care for her animals at home. Issues such as these keep patients from connecting in a positive way to their environments and plans of care.

Then there was Barbara, an 86-year-old who was a ward of the state. Barbara had a Case Manager who followed her care and made many healthcare decisions that impacted her physical and spiritual well-being. Barbara had diabetes, chronic anti-coagulation and peripheral vascular disease. She also developed chronic kidney disease, which ultimately placed her on regular dialysis, even against her will. At age 80, she was tested by a Neuropsychologist, who determined that she was experiencing dementia, but the degree of dementia was never clearly documented in her reports.

Barbara came in with a gangrenous foot, and her state Case Manager considered her to be an endangered adult and filed a court order to amputate her leg and save her life. When I visited with Barbara, she seemed extremely coherent and oriented. After she learned who I was, she made it abundantly clear that she was one of Jehovah's Witnesses and did not want to receive blood products. She described pain in her leg and understood that she needed surgery but was adamant that she not receive blood. After a conversation with her physician, there was no doubt that she would need blood products for this surgery to be successful. Her white-blood-cell count was elevated, and her red-blood-cell count was low. Her international normalized ratio (INR) was 4, and her hemoglobin was at 6.5. In addition to the order to amputate her leg, another court order was filed giving the physician permission to give blood products as needed during surgery. Barbara had made her nurses aware of her personal and religious request not to received blood products, and they were determined not to go against her beliefs and stated desire. The hospital's nurse Case Manager and the state Case Manager were convinced that Barbara had become an adherent of her faith during the time she was determined to have dementia. The staff nurses caring for her requested an ethics committee consult, and a meeting was convened to discuss the case. The basic question was patient autonomy. Another dominate question that kept coming up was since Barbara was a ward of the state, did the state have the right to ignore a patient's religious beliefs, convictions and stated medical directives. Would this constitute a "separation of church and state" issue? The committee, which included Barbara's primary physician, concluded that we were committed to honoring Barbara's wishes not to receive blood. Her physician would write a letter to the state Case Manager offering his professional medical opinion and asking for comfort measures and an Allow Natural Death order to be implemented. (19)

CULTURE-BUILDER

The Pastoral Care provider or Chaplain in a hospital or healthcare setting should be a culture torch-bearer. He or she must become a champion of good HCAHPS scores and more. The Pastoral Care person should be focused on raising the standard of care and compassion for those who are hurting and work to support an environment that is conducive to mental, physical, emotional and spiritual well-being. When an organization collectively fails to become a living, breathing organism that has meaning, purpose and growth, functioning at the highest level and fulfilling its designed purpose, it has lost its way. Pastoral Care strives to build a culture that radiates love, hope, forgiveness, compassion and care. We work to create an environment that accepts patients for who they are and treats them in the way they want to be treated.

There may be those in your organization who need a gentle encouragement to move on to something better. One of my skills involves possessing an eye for those who are living below their potential and need to do that very thing. I've had some experience living below my potential in the past, so it's not that difficult for me to spot a person frustrated with the status quo; a person who may be fed up with what they are doing in the present and looking for something new and exciting to challenge them in the future.

After attending many culture-building sessions, I became a student of Quint Studer's methods of dealing with what he calls high, middle and low performers. (20) Part of the tough talk that managers need to have with those middle and low performers is motivating them to move up or out. As I thought about that concept, I was taken aback by the thought of middle performers who were "stuck" in a position with little chance to move up in the organization. At times, upward movement may be blocked by mid-level managers who themselves need to move up or out. Some high performers and mid-level managers need to move on to specialized fields such as advance practice nurses (APNs) and certified registered nurse anesthetists (CRNAs) or advance into administrative roles such as Chief Nursing Officer (CNO) or perhaps even go on to medical school or other specialized training. "Standing pat" with what they are currently doing will not catapult them in any way toward meeting their professional goals. These employees are bright, astute and articulate, and it is apparent they feel "trapped" and need to move on to a new challenge. I like being a supportive encourager for them in that process.

Then there are the middle performers who truly are disillusioned, bored and feeling more "stuck" by the day, not knowing how or when to make their next move. They probably work well with the people around them, but there is nothing happening that they find fulfilling. At times, I see some of them that will leap over the high performers and enter an advanced healthcare profession, such as those mentioned previously. More often than not, they find a different path that is less obstructed. When high performers block the way of middle performers moving up in the organization, someone needs to move over.

While leadership development initiatives serve to introduce a new cultural dynamic to Administration and mid-level managers, often, it takes some time for meaningful change to occur throughout the whole hospital or system. Pastoral Care providers are a wonderful resource and can become your change agents for a better culture.

PHYSICIAN'S PARACLETE

The word "paraclete" is of Greek origin. A paraclete is one who comes alongside. In the New Testament, Jesus used the verb paraclethesontai (παρακληθήσονται), traditionally interpreted as "to be comforted." The text also may be translated as being in the vocative case, as well as the traditionally interpreted nominative case. In the vocative case, "paraclethesontai," takes on connotations of "are going to summon" or "will be breaking off." Thus, a paraclete may be described as "the summoner" or "the one who makes free."

There have been several occasions when I have had the opportunity to come alongside a physician with words of encouragement after he or she had worked so hard to prolong life, only to fail. The physician's spirit slumps, and he or she starts thinking about things that could have been done differently. Death is a poignant reminder that physicians are human and that, at times, it does not matter what the healthcare team does. People die, despite all the team's efforts. I will never forget a young man who had infection in his heart and how he pleaded with his Cardiologist to save him. As he lay dying, I was present as his physician came into the room. I noticed tears in the physician's eyes as the patient kept pleading for his intervention. "But doctor, isn't there something you can do? I have a wife and daughter," the young husband and father said. After that event, I spoke with the physician and told him that I admired his compassion and all that he did to help this patient. He said, "Chaplain, I feel so helpless. I couldn't do a thing for this man." My encouragement for him was to keep up the compassionate care, knowing full well that he will not save them all, but it was clear to me that his compassionate care and honed medical skills would allow him to help many throughout his career.

Another event I will never forget involved a Cardiovascular surgeon. The patient was scheduled for coronary artery bypass graft surgery, and, early in the morning on the day of his surgery, I arrived to do a spiritual assessment. During our conversation, he told me that he had a feeling that he was not going to survive the operation. I said, "Not going to survive? Tell me more about that." He replied, "It's O.K., because I have lived a good life, and I'm O.K. either way." I'm always curious about such remarks and take them seriously, so I asked for him to tell me more. He said, "Well, you know, Chaplain, there are just some things that a person knows inwardly. You don't know how you know them, you just do." Normally, I would alert the surgeon about comments of this type from a patient, but I was paged away to another Pastoral Care need and was unable to do so before he was taken back to the operating room. Before I left the patient, I assured him that he had a wonderful team working with him and that we were going to keep his family updated throughout the case. In a deeply holy moment, knowing that this could very well be his last moments on Earth, I also told him my prayers were with him. Normally, the mention of prayer will invoke a response of some kind, ranging from the patient requesting a prayer to a simple, "Thank you, I need all the prayers I can get." He simply thanked me. I also asked him if there were any other feelings churning inside that he wanted to talk about. A smile came across his face, and he said, "I'm going to be O.K., no matter what." He died on the operating table, and the surgeon was devastated. After being present with the family for some time, I returned to the operating room only to find the surgeon sitting hunched over in a chair, with his elbows resting on his knees and his face buried in his hands. I gently placed a hand on his shoulder. He lowered his hands from his face to see who had touched him, and I said, "Doc, I know that this is very difficult, but I want you to know that this patient knew he wasn't going to survive this surgery." A look of surprise transformed his somber countenance, as I commenced to tell him about my pre-operative conversation and spiritual assessment with the patient. It is essential for a Pastoral Care provider to come alongside physicians and other inter-disciplinary team members in times like these.

EMPLOYEES' K'HILA K'DOSHA

"K'hila K'dosha" is a Hebrew concept that means "sacred community." It is best exemplified when those in healthcare go through a common experience together, such as a major mass-casualty event, in which everyone had to pull together as a synchronized unit honoring, respecting and caring for each other, both personally and professionally. Something magically happens when a group of people caught in an event beyond their control steps up to meet the demands imposed upon them. The Hurricane Katrina disaster, ice storms, tornadoes and other events are prime examples of times when many in our healthcare system have pulled together for the common good. We in healthcare are action-driven, and when we "ramp it up," things happen – lives are saved and physical, spiritual and emotional needs are met. Pastoral Care providers play a key role in recognizing that dynamic and bringing it to a memorialized conclusion. Often it will be a more spontaneous celebration, whereby everyone can join in a victory song. On the other hand, though, when the outcome is not so joyous, Pastoral Care providers also can pull the healthcare troops together for lament and closure. A sacred community is an environment in which its members can be themselves and express themselves openly and freely, without fear of reprisals.

Our healthcare system has employed upwards of 2,200 staff in the past. When we experience the death of an employee, physician or administrator, a notification of the death is sent out by e-mail to all employees. The notification includes a photo of the departed colleague and specific arrangement information. It also is posted prominently in each nursing unit for employees who do not have access to e-mail. A Reflections Book is placed in the chapel, so employees can experience the quiet solitude found in that spiritual setting and write their words of condolence to the family. Within the notification to staff, is a reminder that if employees go to write in the Reflections Book and find that someone else is writing when they arrive, the person arriving should do the writer the courtesy of giving him or her the space to be alone with his or her thoughts. What I appreciate about this venue of processing a death is that staff can come to the chapel on their own time, and they deeply appreciate that option. For those who cannot attend a memorial service or visitation due to their schedules, this provides a wonderful way for them to process their loss in an appropriate setting, as they reflect upon the life and service of a colleague or valued employee.

Presenting the Reflections Book to scores of families has provided me with a highly effective way to engage them in their time of loss and to convey the healthcare system's deep appreciation for all the times they have shared their loved ones with us. I have seen many tears flow down the cheeks of family members as they receive the book and read what others have written. I have heard family members say how much their loved ones enjoyed their work and how much the staff meant to them. Normally, I will present the Reflections Book to the family. However, there are times when I will have our CEO, COO or other administrative leadership present it. If a physician dies, I usually will present the Reflections Book to his or her spouse on behalf of the employees who have worked with that physician. I would encourage any healthcare system that does not have some method for staff to process such losses to adopt a process that fits its employees and culture.

ADMINISTRATION

It seems like most hospitals and healthcare systems that have Pastoral Care teams underutilize them. This is due, in part, to administrators not knowing the potential of a well-trained Pastoral Care team. But another factor is that Chaplains often fail to take the initiative to demonstrate their department's potential. A certified Pastoral Care provider or Chaplain will have bachelor's and master's degrees, as well as up to 1,600 hours of Clinical Pastoral Education training. The following is a quote from a hospital administrator about certified Chaplains. The administrator explains that certification is supported at by the large health system for which he works, due to "the level of competence that comes with being a professional Chaplain, in a range of ways. (21) Their education and training gives them the skills to integrate spiritual care with disciplines like Psychology, Sociology and Ethics. They have knowledge of best practices and a deeper appreciation of the needs of patients. They also have a deep self-understanding of their own capabilities and limits." A Chaplain who effectively utilizes skills taught in the art of

Pastoral Care can calm angry patients, helping them get back in sync with a plan of care, head off potential litigation and raise the overall patient satisfaction.

BRIDGE TO THE COMMUNITY

The community or region that your hospital or healthcare system serves will benefit from your providing Pastoral Care services. Not only does it impact an institution's public image, it comforts the general public to know that there is someone on staff whose job is to maintain high moral, ethical and spiritual standards. That being said, there are people in every profession who do not rise to that public expectation. Pastoral Care providers or Chaplains can reflect back to Administration that which is being perceived in the community. Just as Clinical Pastoral Education students glean insights from times when their peer group members "hold up a mirror" to show them how their ministry is perceived, Administration can glean much from the feedback a Pastoral Care provider shares with his or her administrative team.

ADDITIONAL COMMENTS

In this chapter, we have observed some of the ways Pastoral Care services reach out to support and encourage patients, families, staff, physicians, administrators and the community as they experience challenging events. Having Pastoral Care in a hospital or healthcare system will add a great deal of depth to the care and compassion being delivered to those who are hurting and in search of healing. Pastoral Care providers can blaze the trail in areas where others fear to tread. In the midst of crisis situations, their emotional control can have a calming effect on others. Knowing the Self in a dynamic way and utilizing appropriate pastoral authority will earn the respect of many members of the healthcare teams, as well as patients and their families, all of whom may be struggling to find a measure of peace during tumultuous times. CPE students under my supervision often are encouraged not to let their heart rates rise any higher than those of the people involved in the situation at hand. Sometimes, that can be a real challenge for them, but appropriate utilization of Pastoral Care skills makes it possible.

Being present for a patient and going where they need to go is entirely different from being guided by a personal agenda or bias, in which case, there is great potential to miss the real need, perhaps "by a million miles." Being available for patients and going where they need to go in conversation is an art that requires the artist to utilize a unique set of skills and to know the correct time to use them. The manner in which this objective is accomplished depends on the Pastoral Care provider. If a Chaplain is present to help facilitate a patient's inner processing and healing through the utilization of specific skills, then patients stand a much better chance of aligning with their plans of care and becoming synchronized in body, mind and spirit.

As I begin each CPE unit, I remind students that I do not expect them to know what they have come to learn – a phrase that one of my past CPE supervisors shared with me. Below is a graph that I have CPE students use at the beginning of the unit to help them plot where they are with cognitive, affective, "being" and "doing" issues, as they interact with patients, family, staff, physicians and others. They plot themselves on the graph at the beginning and again at the end of the unit, so that they can visually measure their progress. This has proven to be a productive visual aid for them.

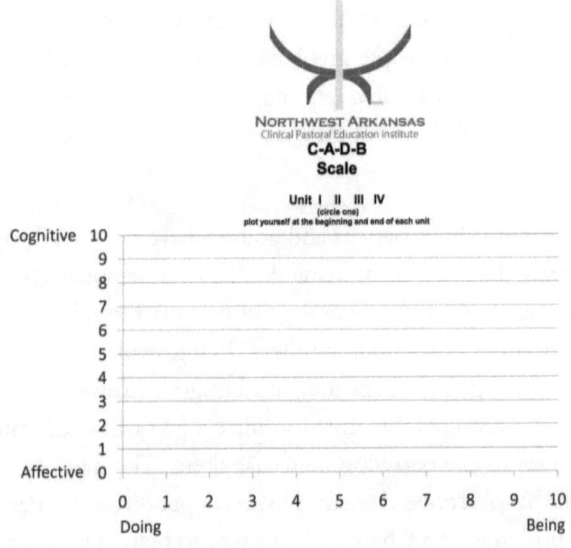

Finally, good pastoral presence and Pastoral Care is an asset to any hospital or healthcare system, no matter the size. Those who currently are in the "curing" mindset of treating disease processes and not as concerned about "healing" can revitalize their services to basic human needs through offering pastoral presence to those in need.

Chapter Four – Corporate Acquisitions

This is the most compelling chapter for me to write. It strikes at the core of what mid-level management and healthcare staff experience during corporate acquisitions. While corporate strategists may be rejoicing in a new acquisition and what it means for their corporate successes, many mid-level managers, supervisors, physicians and employees are being more deeply affected, and not always in a positive manner. With CEO changes coming every 2-4 years and constant corporate mandates trickling down, equilibrium and cultural health in hospitals and healthcare systems is difficult to maintain. Organizations need to allow appropriate time for their people to process and adjust to major changes. My experiences with corporate change during the past 30 years provided the impetus for creating a diagram of stages encountered by mid-level management and other staff during such paradigm shifts. Not only will I attempt to identify feelings and behaviors demonstrated by staff, I will also attempt to reflect on pastoral presence and its effectiveness in each phase.

The following are my personal observations from some of my first-hand experiences with corporate acquisitions over the years. Each one has provided an opportunity for me to observe and assess the processes staff experienced. I firmly believe that good pastoral presence and knowledge of each phase will help people adjust and stay focused on their roles, as the acquisition moves along.

Grand Rapids Public Schools & Education Management Corporation:

In the late 1980s, the Job Corp Center of Grand Rapids, Mich., was being managed on a contractual basis by the Grand Rapids Public School System. In early 1989, the contract was bought by Education Management Corporation (EMC) of Pittsburgh, Pa., and an administration change was imminent for that Center. My employment as a vocational and academic counselor began while the Center was still under the public school's management, and I maintained my position through the transition and for several months into Education Management Corporation's contract.

As the rumors of contract ownership and administration change began, the buzz at the Center was clearly felt by everyone. Administration under the public school contract knew that they would need to seek other positions within the school system. Most of the remaining staff of resident advisers, teachers and counselors hoped to stay employed with the new owners. Once Education Management Corporation (EMC) was awarded the new contract, staff began asking about them and researching their history and reputation. It was their attempt at getting a feel for what brand of leadership the new administration would bring and what would be required of them if they were to remain employed at the Center.

One of the main issues that surfaced early on was EMC potentially requiring employees hired by the school to go through a formal interview process to maintain their positions. In essence, they would go through the hiring process once again to keep their jobs. This requirement served many practical purposes in that it provided EMC an opportunity to assess qualifications, competencies and skills. It also provided existing employees the opportunity to assess their desire to stay or make a move. As it turned out, all of public school administration assigned to the Center took positions within the school system, and the rest of staff interviewed by EMC continued in their positions. While under the Grand Rapids Public School contract, Western Michigan University Education Department served as consultants to Job Corp Center staff during the transition. They would provide didactics on issues relevant to the Job Corp environment, and they also assisted in preparing staff, to some degree, for the upcoming contract and leadership changes.

As EMC began to fulfill its contractual agreement, a new Executive Director was named. It seemed to me that the EMC leadership made little effort to get a feel for the existing culture of the Center prior to his arrival. Since the new Executive Director had some previous experience in a Job Corps Center, Their thought may have been that he would know the culture and make the changes necessary for the center to be productive and profitable.

After learning whom the new contract holder would be, we were given very little information about Education Management Corporation and how they were structured on the corporate level and what an organization chart looked like in their contracted centers. It was a huge learning curve for those who remained to work at the Center. As I look back at that experience, it would have gone much smoother if EMC would have held meetings that allowed existing employees to process frustration with the past administration and express what they hoped for in this new relationship. Had they shared a realistic picture of EMC with staff and answered questions in a transparent manner, some of those who left may have stayed and those who did stay, along with the students currently enrolled, might have experienced a better transition.

As it turned out, when the new Executive Director was named, rumors began to surface by those who knew his past record at other Centers. He immediately began to initiate change and a new culture, but staff and students knew quickly that he was not the right fit for the Center. After a few months in his position, many of the students refused to return to the Center after a holiday break. His style of management needed to change, or a new Executive Director search would be required. While a strong accountability culture was certainly needed for those inner-city students, his style of autocratic leadership triggered a negative response from the very people he was there to serve. As his style of leadership continued to be challenged, he became more and more defensive. Many good staff members lost their positions because they would personally challenge his leadership style. Ultimately, he was replaced by a new Executive Director, who had much greater success. He had the experience and ability to work relationally with not only the corporate leadership but also the administration, staff and students at the Center.

Quorum Health Resources (QHR)

In early 2000, I was hired as a staff Chaplain for Northwest Health System, and 30 days later I was promoted to Director of Pastoral Care for the system. Quorum Health Resources of Brentwood, Tenn., a for-profit entity managing hospitals, had purchased Springdale Memorial Hospital in Springdale, Ark., and Bates Medical Center of Bentonville, Arkansas. Both hospitals were previously not-for-profit entities so going from ownership by a locally controlled entity with an active, community-based Board of Trustees to a Wall Street-traded corporation was challenging for staff, physicians and all of Northwest Arkansas. All eyes were focused on the results. The Community Care Foundation was established to manage the proceeds from the sale. This Foundation has become a valuable source of funding for many non-profit entities throughout Northwest Arkansas. The Board of Trustees at each acquired hospital lost their fiduciary responsibilities they had known in the past and became an advisory board to the new owners.

In addition to growing a corporation, a primary objective for this new acquisition was to create greater profitability and mold the system into a for-profit model of healthcare delivery. The new administration implemented many changes early on, and in the alignment process, several programs and positions were eliminated as cost-saving measures. It didn't take long for staff to assess the new CEO and identify him as the "hatchet man" sent from corporate headquarters to "slash and burn."

Needless to say, staff, physicians and the community experienced some shock over such drastic measures. Bill

89

Bradley, the second CEO under Quorum ownership actually had ties to the area and had been in corporate healthcare for many years. After a long career in corporate healthcare, which took him many places, he desired to move closer to his roots here in Northwest Arkansas. He took over as CEO, bringing to us a wealth of leadership experience. Bill was gifted at being relational, creating stability, growing product lines and finding profitability for our system. In casual conversation one day, he told me that when he took over, the system was on the verge of being closed but that things were turning around. And turn around it did. As we experienced his leadership, it was abundantly clear that it was his vision, hard work and ability to keep staff informed that contributed greatly to his success. One could tell he was where he wanted to be, and he exuded confidence in his leadership decisions. In the short time he was with us, he truly gained the respect of patients, staff, physicians and the community.

Triad Hospitals Inc.

In the fall of 2000 (as reported in the Oct. 30, 2000, edition of Weekly Corporate Growth Report), (22) Triad Hospitals, Inc. of Plano, Texas, agreed to purchase Quorum Health Resources. Triad was a new, upstart company representing what was once the Hospital Corporation of America (HCA) Pacific Group. Many of Triad's leadership team had experience with Quorum and Tenet Healthcare in managing hospitals and healthcare systems. Triad's senior leadership seemed to possess a democratic, participative leadership style. Early on in their short-lived history, it was not uncommon for the corporate CEO to visit our system meeting with Administration and our mid-level management team in an open-forum style. They wanted to hear from us as they worked to mold this new corporation, and we felt empowered to do our jobs without too much micro-managing at the mid-level. The exchange of information about the company was free-flowing. When there were major changes on the horizon, we were informed expeditiously and as thoroughly as could be done at the time. Triad's senior management team brought a collective wealth of experience that was easily recognized by staff and physicians. It seemed as though their mantra for this new corporation was to take the best of what they had gleaned over the years and mold it into their matrix. It seemed as though they were also searching for a culture that would be the "gold standard" for the healthcare industry. Their openness to new ideas and best practices was a breath of fresh air to our system. Mid-level managers felt they were a part of something new and innovative, and that gave them purpose and drive.

Our CEO continued to show us his appreciation for our dedicated work by authorizing bonuses, team-building trips and even in times when the balance sheet could not support end-of-year bonuses, each director was given a cheesecake as a token of appreciation. CEOs should remember that not enough can be said for this type of leadership and acts of appreciation. Then word came that Bill Bradley was leaving to be the CEO of our competitor just a few miles down the road. This news was devastating and created another loss in our system that needed to be grieved, since this CEO was so well-liked and had done so many good things for the system. He had won our hearts. Why was he leaving us? The move was so swift that we had very little closure time. Triad wasted very little time naming an interim CEO, who later took on the job as our system CEO. They tried to involve us in the process as much as possible, but we actually didn't have much input. The CEO who took over had been tagged for a new acquisition in a nearby city but that acquisition did not materialize so Triad moved him up the road to us. While he did some good things for the system, he did not have the same vested interest as the previous CEO, and most people sensed it.

A year or two after the CEO change, Triad announced that it was selling to Community Health Systems, and the world we knew was changing yet again. The directors were summoned to the Board Room, and the CEO announced the sale to us. It threw us into another dilemma, and the department directors were left to process more change. We were starting to get the picture of corporate-run healthcare, which seemed to be fraught with change and more change. We did not know if our CEO would remain with us or move on. Once again, we had many unanswered questions and very little closure. I had the feeling that a new leadership team would be taking over, much like what happens when a senior pastor moves to a new congregation and brings along his ministry team.

Community Health Systems (CHS)

In the spring of 2007 (as reported in MarketWatch, on March 19, 2007), Community Health Systems agreed to buy Triad Hospitals. (23) After the sale, our CEO stayed with us for only a few months. On the day his resignation was announced at a directors' meeting, his comment to me as he walked forward to tell us of his resignation was, "Buy low and sell high!" We were given another interim CEO until CHS could do a national search for the right person. The CHS corporate management style seemed to be less open than that of Triad. Corporate leadership did not keep us routinely updated, but an occasional division CEO visit would occur. Once again, mid-level managers and others in our system were left wondering what would happen next. We were truly in a state of flux for a year, as we awaited corporate direction. Much of this lag time was due to the fact that, with this acquisition, CHS had doubled in size. They, too, wanted to take the best of both corporations and build a better corporate entity. It actually took nearly three years to start hearing positive affirmation from staff about the help that CHS Corporate was able to provide our system.

A new CEO was hired, and less than a year later, in March 2010, our CEO and CFO resigned their positions, creating, yet again, a jarring loss for the system. In the past 15 years, our system has had nine CEOs and more than 11 CFOs. The leadership shifts alone become wearisome to staff and physicians alike. It seems like every new CEO comes on board with his or her idea of how best to lead the system forward to a positive community reputation, cutting-edge services and profitability. Most of our CEOs have had to make drastic cuts to accommodate soft volumes and rising bad-debt expenses, due to the rapid growth in the number of uninsured patients. Stabilization for the system definitely has been needed but as yet has been so elusive. It is interesting that the two top-performing hospitals in CHS have CEOs who each have been with their hospital for nearly 20 years. It goes without saying that stability in Administration contributes to the creation of high-performing hospitals.

Enough can't be said about how a CEO's personality and leadership style affect his or her team. CEO styles are as varied as personality types. Some have the experience and ability to empower people and change culture quickly, while others attempt to wield their power to personal ends. Leadership styles among CEOs range from laissez faire to autocratic. There are upward-focused CEOs who feel they have much to prove in the corporate environment, and personal advancement becomes their primary objective. On the other hand, there also are seasoned CEOs who have the ability to steer the canoe effectively to avoid obstacles in the healthcare stream. No matter what, a CEO who cares about people as much as he does about numbers will make a valuable mark on the team he leads and the community they serve together.

When Northwest Health System was purchased by CHS, all many directors wanted to do was to "fly under the radar." We focused on our departments and stayed clear of what was going on in Administration. Occasionally, we would ask each other for the latest information on where we were headed, but, of course, no one actually knew. For most of us mid-level managers, it took as long as three years before we began to feel any sense of integration. I'm sure that many of the emotional and behavioral components mentioned in each phase of the diagram below contributed to that lengthy process. We all desired to become a cohesive team once again, but it just wasn't happening very fast at all. It was a huge learning curve for most of us, and as the corporate transplants started coming into our system, it took time to learn their perspectives and leadership styles.

The presence of Pastoral Care during corporate healthcare acquisitions can be a great benefit to mid-level managers and staff. Not only are Pastoral Care professionals trained to be present for individuals in crisis, they also know that in all transitions of life and work, there are times when employees, physicians, managers and administration need to vent, lament and grieve. While Pastoral Care is also impacted by corporate change, a Pastoral Care provider can provide the impetus for a smoother and more productive transition. While some Pastoral Care staff may get caught up in the tide of emotion, along with others, the trained and experienced ones will know how to remain objective. A Pastoral Care professional must remain as neutral as possible. That will allow a Pastoral Care provider to ask some of the more difficult questions that others only wish they could ask of corporate leadership. The questions have no hidden agenda, only the desire to obtain clarification on key matters affecting all involved.

Not only does a Pastoral Care provider advocate for the patient and family, they also become an advocate for clear communication and information during times of transition. Holding leadership accountable for promises made may be the exact type of thing you would need to speak to on behalf of mid-level management and employees. It takes Pastoral Care leaders who are secure in their pastoral authority to stand up for what is right. Church history is replete with the likes of Deitrich Bonhoeffer, the Lutheran Pastor who, in the 1930s and 1940s stood up and fought the rising tide of

National Socialism (and the Nazi Party). Surely he and others have taught us a valuable lesson: to be the voice for the many. There is a lesson to be learned about knowing and understanding one's environment and how it is being impacted by an event. The possibility that a Pastoral Care provider's position may be lost in the acquisition should never deter him or her from "standing in the gap." Being available and providing pastoral presence is essential in times of change and transition.

ADJUSTMENT PHASES FOR ACQUIRED HOSPITAL STAFF

After an acquisition, it takes time, patience and a willingness to face tough challenges to get a hospital or healthcare system to live up to its potential. As managers and employees move from phase to phase, keep in mind that the end result of the process should be a cohesive team that is focused on doing their best for the patient and running a hospital as effectively and efficiently as possible. We should never lose sight of who we are there to serve – the patient. Mid-level managers informed of these phases will have a more positive effect on the staff under their leadership. When the coach is having a tough time personally, the players pick up on it. A coach who keeps faith in the players during a game, in which the team is several points behind, motivates the team immensely. A leader's personal faith in his or her team and ability to keep them focused on the mission before them will keep hope alive. Faithful leadership will help staff "keep on keeping on" and hold strong to the belief that, at any moment, the tide will turn, and the victory will be sweet.

As a freshman in high school, I received some encouraging words that I will always remember. They came from my track coach, Mike Frey, as I was running the mile event at a track meet in Liberty, Ill. I was in fourth place, with two laps to go. Coach Frey pointed to the guy several paces ahead of me and said, just focus on passing him. With that encouragement, I set my mind to do just that and ended up taking third place in the event. The life lesson that I gleaned from that comment was to focus on that which lies directly in front of me. Do what I can today, because tomorrow will have a new set of challenges. Getting too global during a major event like an acquisition will divide perspective and draw focus away from the task at hand. If I had pushed myself to win first place during that track event, I would have fallen in exhaustion and not placed at all. During an acquisition, Pastoral Care providers should keep focused on the phase they are experiencing in the moment and realize that there is a momentum pushing the event down the course to a designated finish. The best we can do is to challenge ourselves to believe in what we are doing and trust the process.

Another awareness of personal dynamics surfaced in me during these corporate acquisitions. It had to do with my father's leadership style and its impact on our sibling group – all nine of us. He would not allow us to question his authority or decisions. If we did, it was met with harsh responses and sometimes punishment. I learned to keep my mouth shut in his presence, when, deep inside, I wanted to question things or offer my opinion. It took me a long time to be able to ask clarifying questions – or questions of any kind, for that matter – without slipping back into the inhibiting fear I had experienced from my father. However, as I began asking questions during our acquisition meetings, staff would come up to me and convey their thankfulness for my asking such questions, as they were too afraid to do so. As it took time for me to free myself from that inhibited feeling, it also takes time for those being acquired to acclimate to a new parent company. The diagram that follows illustrates various adjustment phases that mid-level managers and staff may experience during acquisitions. This model may also fit major changes encountered in other corporate settings outside healthcare. Each phase in this diagram illustrates the observed experiences and behaviors of Administration, mid-level management and staff when Triad Hospitals (i.e., Northwest Health System) was purchased by Community Health Systems in 2007. Each phase is identified by using XY coordinates in uppercase and lowercase. Uppercase coordinates represent dominance, while the lowercase letter represents recessive or subordinate traits. The positioning of uppercase and lowercase letters signifies the order of dominance.

While most Pastoral Care providers are versed in one therapy or another, Cognitive Behavior Therapy (CBT), which stems from Albert Ellis' Rational Emotive Behavior Therapy (REBT) gave me a good handle on assessing individuals and groups in each phase. CBT often is used in individual therapy, as well as in group settings, and the techniques adapted for self-help applications. Some clinicians and researchers are more cognitively oriented (e.g. cognitive restructuring), while others are more behaviorally oriented (in vivo exposure therapy). Other interventions combine both (e.g. imaginal exposure therapy). (24) (25) CBT was primarily developed through a merging of behavior therapy with cognitive therapy. While rooted in rather different theories, these two traditions found common ground in focusing on the "here and now," and on alleviating symptoms. (26) There are observable emotions and behaviors noted in each phase, as well as a brief reflection on how Pastoral Care and presence, much of which I provided, reached out to those impacted.

It is also important to note that some phases are completed by legal finality. Other phases reach completion in a relatively short period of time. And then there are those phases that require a much longer period of time for completion to occur. Since each employee's personality differs, the level of personal impact in each phase and the progression from one phase to another may not result in everyone being "on board" as the majority move into the next phase. There will be stragglers, so "leaving the 99 to rescue the one" may be the order of the day for the Pastoral Care provider. Also, keep in mind that vacillation between phases occurred. To the astute observer, it will become clear when a new phase has emerged. Sensing phase completion comes from listening closely to the questions posed and comments made along the way. It is key to stay tuned to behaviors demonstrated by the majority of managers and employees, as well as staying in tune with the overall spirit of the organization.

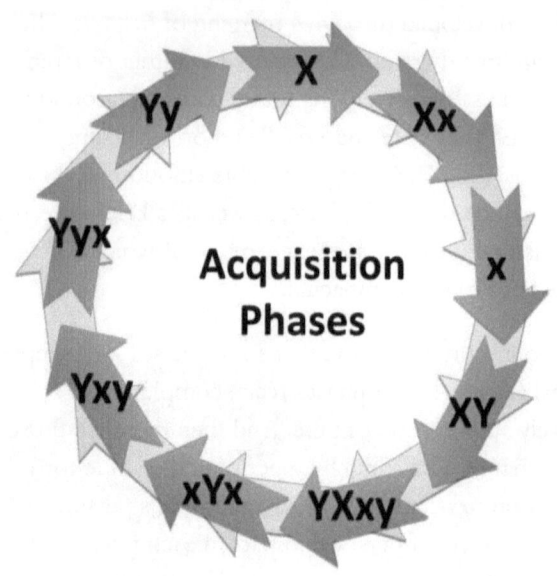

LEGEND:

X = Triad and NHS Administration

x = mid-level managers/directors

Y = CHS and NHS Administration

y = mid-level managers/directors

PROCESSING PHASES:

X = Impact Phase

Xx = Dissemination Phase

x = Disassociating Phase

XY = Transitional Phase

YXxy = Official Phase

xYy = Resistance/Individuation Phase

Yxy = Positioning Phase

Yyx = Integration/Assimilation Phase

Yy = Acculturated/Cohesive Phase

X = Impact Phase

Coordinate positioning note: This phase focuses on Triad
and our NHS administrative team and it occurs when Wall
Street news meets Main Street. Information that may have
been swirling for some time finally arrives at the front door
of the hospital or healthcare system, and rumors of being
purchased by another corporation (if they existed) are now
confirmed. Those who follow Security and Exchange
Commission articles and track other financial media outlets
such as MarketWatch already may have had a "heads up" on
this acquisition, but in our situation, the majority of us had
no clue. It took most of us totally by surprise. Once it is out,
the news of an acquisition travels at Facebook speed through
the ranks of both the purchased entity and the one acquiring
it. Local competitors will start asking questions and
positioning themselves for new challenges as they learn of it.

Once the news reaches the local hospital or healthcare
system that is being acquired, the CEO and administrative
team begin processing a new reality, and wheels start turning.
The effect of the acquisition on their current positions and

future livelihoods will start to sink in. Making sure they can align themselves with the new owners is vital. If the hospital or healthcare system being acquired is community-owned, the whole hospital or system will be swept into a very foreign corporate environment. Greater sensitivity and patience are needed on both sides when this is the case.

BEHAVIORS:

The news of Northwest Health System's acquisition left many of us stunned. It generated reactions ranging from tears to head-shaking frustration. We had put a lot of energy into getting a culture established that would catapult us to the top. We were enjoying a cohesive team spirit between Administration, mid-level management, physicians and staff prior to the acquisition. Of course, there were those who appeared outwardly unfazed throughout the process, although they processed the change inwardly. As I visited with directors and others, they identified feelings of fear, frustration, anger, betrayal, alienation, loss, detachment, disillusionment, etc. Loss certainly catapults a person into the grief process. As in the impact stage of grief, I heard questions and statements such as, "What will we do now?" "I heard the rumors, but I just can't believe it happened again!" "Where do we go from here?" We all attempted to keep smiles on our faces, but it was obvious that sometimes, the smiles merely masked many of the aforementioned feelings. As mentioned earlier, our system has had nine CEOs and more than 11 CFOs in the past 15 years.

PASTORAL FOCUS:

The multiple leadership changes became wearisome and compounded mid-level managers' ability to create trust in Administration. Much of my pastoral presence during this phase mirrored the presence provided during the impact stage of grief. There was the befuddled and consternated shaking of heads and the remarks of, "Here we go again," that I witnessed so often. During this time, I remembered that it's not what we say to the affected people that makes a difference, it's being there for them and allowing them to go where they need to go that can make all the difference in the world. Allowing them opportunity to identify and name the feelings that churn inside gives them ownership of those feelings. Processing them up and out will allow that person to reconnect to his or her purpose more quickly, without harboring feelings inside that can rob them of focus. It is important to remember that Pastoral Care providers are there for the whole hospital or system, from the top down. Be present for those totally frustrated and avoid using "us vs. them" themes.

Some directors of Pastoral Care answer directly to the CEO, while others answer to other administrative team members. No matter whom the Pastoral Care Director reports to, Administration can use good pastoral presence, too. Intentionally checking in on them as they do their processing is important and appreciated. Directors of Pastoral Care who have very little personal contact with their CEO and Administration will miss out on a chance to provide good Pastoral Care and presence. For the administrative team that is acquiring another hospital or healthcare system, my recommendation is that directors of Pastoral Care or the Pastoral Care provider start establishing a rapport early on in the process. The Pastoral Care Director could be the bridge that administration needs to connect them to their newly acquired mid-level management, employees, physicians and community. Administrators are people who carry a heavy load at times and letting them know what Pastoral Care professionals are observing, hearing and perceiving can be valuable information. Conveying what you hear in the community and from area clergy as they visit patients in the hospital gives Administration a take on how the acquisition is being perceived and accepted.

Xx = Dissemination Phase

Coordinate positioning note: Information being disseminated from Triad's corporate office by our system CEO to mid-level managers and/or directors. This phase involves NHS Administration and its management team. On a Friday afternoon in the early spring of 2007, our mid-level managers were summoned to a meeting in the Administrative Conference Room. After getting off the phone with corporate leadership, our CEO came in to inform us that we had new owners. The mid-level management of our healthcare system under Triad was a cohesive team, and when the announcement was made, the room was filled with many strong emotions – some of which ran quite deep. A few managers sat there with stoic expressions on their faces. It was like a two-ton boulder had been thrown into a half-acre farm pond … again. The prevailing question around the conference table was, "Where do we go from here?" As other questions poured out, it became clear from the tones of voice used by those who were speaking that strong feelings had been triggered.

The CEO attempted to lay out for us what he thought would take place, but we all knew that this was "the end of the line" for the culture we were working so hard to build. Our "ownership" was going to slip away, and someone else would present us with a new culture to champion. Feelings of anger and fear were present. Our time, energy and talents had been poured into our effort to be the best we could be. Fear of the unknown and an overwhelming loss of direction became the guiding forces for what once has been a relational and functional team. The following questions were posed to our CEO:

- "Was it a friendly takeover or just another corporate deal?"
- "What's next for us?"
- "In this time of transition, who has the answers, and who will be communicating with us?"
- "How will we be informed of upcoming changes?"
- "How much corporate 'shuffle' will be going on?"
- "Why were we sold?"

Some of the more direct questions included:

- "Whose pockets are being lined, and how much are the key players walking away with?"
- "What is the reputation of our new owners?"
- "Who among Administration will stay, and who will go?"
- "Why didn't anyone ask us if we wanted to be sold?"

After the news settled in a bit, the CEO left the room, and we began processing even more. There were words of encouragement to shore everyone and rally the team once again, because we knew we were a good team who had come through a lot together. Affirmations of each other's contributions to the team were expressed.

As I reflect on my own history with those four little words, "We have new owners," I believe strongly that it is important for a CEO to provide opportunity for those present to ask questions as they begin to process the event. If there is a question posed for which they do not have an answer, most people can accept, "I don't know." Once a rock is thrown into a pond, the ripple effects begin. And if the waters already were choppy, the ripples may not be as easily distinguishable. If our healthcare system had been in a state of flux or turmoil prior to the news of the acquisition, the impact may not have been as shocking. However, for us the opposite was true, and the impact was like a major earthquake, followed by a tsunami. Ripples will keep coming, and sometimes we fail to realize how far they can reach. People thousands of miles away may feel some effects, as the news disseminates. Text messages, Facebook, and all electronic media will be abuzz, for sure. A day after this meeting, a Director of Pastoral Care from a healthcare system 200 miles away called to get an update.

As we processed the news, it was now our turn to officially break the news to our staff, and many of the questions and dynamics already mentioned were present. We kept our staff focused on what they were here to do – care for our patients. Keeping them focused does not mean they won't have many more questions and wonder how you are taking the news. We were all as positive as we could be and, due to our shared experience with a past acquisition, we were somewhat experienced at navigating through this territory.

BEHAVIORS:

Feelings ran strong during the meeting, as I observed some shaking their heads in disbelief. There was a collective exhale, and I heard someone say, "Not again!" When a team that has such a high degree of cohesiveness and is "buzzing along" hears such news, often, the "brakes" are applied quite abruptly. We wanted to protect what we had, and our sense of pride was being stripped away. We knew we were a tenacious, stalwart, prideful and possessive bunch, and we were not ready to give up without a fight. Listening to comments and questions and observing body language from the mid-level management team tells a lot about team cohesiveness. Words of encouragement could be heard from various team members, as they thought about all they had worked so hard to create. "We are a good team and have worked hard to get where we are today!" "We will just have to pull together, and we will get through this."

PASTORAL FOCUS:

As the Director of Pastoral Care, I knew this was a time when the staff needed me, and I needed to be present for them in a new way until we found our way together through this acquisition. Our team needed a good listener as they lamented. It was indeed my intent to keep my ears, eyes and heart open during this phase.

Noting who was absent from the meeting was important to me, since I wanted to follow up with them later to check in with them about the acquisition. Observing those who just walked away without saying a word and seeking them out later for more processing was important as well. Also, I made an attempt to remember those in the meeting who were more emotional, realizing that sometimes this may indicate something else being triggered in them that is not even related to the acquisition announcement. From this time on, in addition to being focused on our Priority of Needs, my role took on some new responsibilities – intentional pastoral presence to mid-level managers. My mind also focused on trying to find ways to include the clinics connected to our healthcare system. Often, they feel disconnected from what is happening and yet, during these times, plenty of Pastoral Care needs are present there as well. There were many people from the community who would stop me and ask what was going on. They wanted assurance that the same level of care that they had experienced in the past would still be provided by the new ownership. I found myself visiting all departments on all campuses, in order to be present for them. With loss, there is grief to be observed and processed.

x = Disassociating Phase

Coordinate positioning note: This phase represents NHS mid-level managers and/or directors finding closure and processing upcoming changes. No sooner had the dissemination phase been experienced than the disassociating phase began. There were some mid- level managers who overlapped Xx and x phases. It took time for the news to sink in, and I observed some of our staff who kept disassociating, even well into the transition and official phases before they could move on. This phase is painful, but necessary, for all the people involved to process the events completely. It is the phase that's all about the closure process, saying "good-bye" to what was and starting to gain enough strength to accept what is yet to come.

Our mid-level management team knew that Administration would change and that the leadership team we once knew would no longer have the same construct. The mid-level managers actually took on quite a bit more leadership responsibility during this phase. To lessen the impact of this phase, some managers drew inward, and others focused more intently on their department and staff, in order to shore them up and prepare them to function at the perceived production level that the new administration and corporation would want from them.

This phase was also a time of personal assessment and decision-making for mid-level management. Do I have the skills that the new corporation will require of me? How will I fit into this new corporation? Is this the opportune time for me to retire? Is this the chance I have been looking for to make a job or career change? What will be expected of me and my staff? Will more work be piled on my plate? The concept of "team" began to unravel, and directors relied more on their own skills to carry them through.

BEHAVIORS:

Mid-level managers and some supervisors experienced strong feelings and demonstrated soul-searching behaviors during this phase, as they continued to process personal and professional questions. In my departmental observations, some staff were astute at picking up on their directors' struggles with processing the issues. As I reflect on that observation, my advice is that directors be careful to keep their processing "under wraps" until it is completed. This can be a challenge for some who process life events more openly than others. Feelings seemed to vacillate between personal confidence and doubt. It is truly a time to settle the question of whether to stay or go. That decision can be a lonely, heart-wrenching process, but each person needs to find peace with his or her answer. From my own experience, I know there will be times when people attempting to answer this question find themselves vacillating. Emotional "winds" bend a person first one direction and then another. As those "winds" buffet, managers and directors, it can be difficult to project an upright and steadfast spirit to your staff. The stress of disassociation is real and cannot be eased by anyone except the person who must endure it. It's a time for deep self-reflection, professional decision-making and asking many questions that can impact family, staff and others.

PASTORAL FOCUS:

This is a difficult phase to process, since there are many unknowns out there, and each change introduces even more. Doing good closure work is essential to moving forward without "baggage" in tow. A new chapter is about to open, and while staff always will remember what was, they also will need to clear the slate for something new. Change can be difficult for many people, and it is even more difficult when several changes are experienced in rapid succession, as many of our mid-level managers knew well. Be patient and present for those making a major decision. Some administrators and mid-level managers may use this disassociating phase to retire. Retiring provides an opportunity to turn yet another change into a celebration. Be present and celebrate this special milestone with them. Sorting through feelings of doubt and trying to imagine in your mind how it's all going to work out requires a lot of mental processing – and often, a step of faith. Affirming a person's worth and value is essential during this phase.

XY = Transition Phase

Coordinate positioning note: X & Y are the key focus at this time. This is the phase in which we were told that the corporate legal team was tying up "loose ends," and CHS was preparing to take ownership. I'm sure there still could have been glitches that would have derailed the transaction, but we all knew that the Securities and Exchange Commission had placed its stamp of approval on it, so that possibility was unlikely. During this phase, I observed staff asking each other in the hallways whether they had heard anything more about the signing of the final papers. We were keenly aware of new faces on campus. When we saw someone we didn't know, we would either stop and introduce ourselves or stop someone we did know and ask who that person was, how they fit in and what position they would hold. We began to wonder who in administration was going to be replaced and with whom? The mental transitions that take place in this phase can be a challenge. As stated earlier, those in the disassociation phase may continue to process some heavy personal and professional options. Speculation by staff was rampant throughout the system, and yet no one really knew anything. The only thing we knew for sure was that things would not look the same in the near future. More questions:

- "Who are those guys?"
- "Who will be our new CEO?"
- "Where's our COO … have you seen him lately?"
- "Who's moving up or out?"
- "Will there be staff reductions?"
- "What will our new face of healthcare look like?"
- "What type of culture will they bring to us?"

BEHAVIORS:

Those still struggling with the earlier dissemination phase were either in the process of looking for a new position or making the decision to remain and get on board with a new team. Managers and staff began guessing what the big picture would look like. Ambiguity, feelings of isolation, questions related to job security and Human Resources-type concerns circulated everywhere.

PASTORAL FOCUS:

Affirming staff's significance was the order of the day. Openly greeting new faces and asking them open-ended questions to gain more information about their position with the new corporate owners was beneficial. Several times, I would introduce myself to those I did not recognize and say, "Hi, I'm C.J., system director for our Pastoral Care … and your name is … ?" "How are you connected with our new owners?" There were many times that the person was not connected at all, only outside consultants doing business related to the transaction. Much of my time directly related to the acquisition was spent assuring staff that no matter who owned us, patient care should be our immediate focus.

YXxy = Official Phase

Coordinate positioning note: Y and X still dominate the focus. In the mindset of x, the NHS mid-level managers, they were still dominant, even though the Y and X had shifted positions. Triad was phasing out, and CHS was in control. The small y managers knew that this acquisition was going to double the size of their corporation. No doubt, CHS corporate headquarters was abuzz with major changes, as well. As the new corporation's leadership worked on figuring out their next move, employees of both corporations experienced their own brand of trying to figure things out. When confirmation finally came that the deal was indeed completed, it was like closing on a house. The papers all had been signed and the real estate agent had turned over the keys. The new owners were empowered to take possession. Staff continued to have questions regarding leadership styles, expectations, compensation, benefits and which members of the past Administration would stay or go. Some in Administration probably already knew in which direction they were headed. We were all anxious to identify corporate personnel – put a face with a name, hopefully in the same manner that Triad had introduced themselves to us. The vibe seemed to be reflected in questions like:

- "Who are they, anyway, and when are they going to introduce themselves to us?"

- "How safe is my position?"
- "Who from our hospital will emerge as a leader in this new structure?"
- "What will change for me as a result of this new entity?"
- "What is their management style, and what culture will they present to us?"
- "How will they better us as a healthcare system?"
- "Will they be as progressive as we were under Triad?"
- "What innovations will they bring?"
- "How much capital will they put into our system?"

BEHAVIORS:

Directors were feeling a sense of relief and excitement as the drama began to subside and a new reality began to set in. Most were ready for it all to be over. While many questions still remained, as noted previously, we wanted to know if our CEO was going to stay on or go. Getting to know the new leadership and processing their style was on our minds. We were anxious for the leadership picture to emerge more clearly.

PASTORAL FOCUS:

Keeping focused on the Priority of Needs structure for the health system, managing the everyday pastoral needs and wondering whether Pastoral Care would be looked on favorably by the new corporation kept me busy. This was a time for me to sit down with my staff and help them process, as well. They needed space and time to work through their own concerns, so they could go forth to be present for others. It was apparent that mid-level managers were in the process of preparing themselves and their departments for this new reality that was about to descend upon them. Staying focused and keeping staff engaged in a positive manner was our focus.

xYy = Resistance/Individuation Phase

Coordinate positioning note: It is apparent that x has not given up its position yet. We were confident that the policies and practices under our former owners were the best ones for our system. Yet Human Resources started sharing new policies and procedures from CHS corporate headquarters, and the changes began. We knew our benefits package under Triad, and staff began wondering how much of that would go away under CHS. We had directors' meetings to roll out the policies, and it took time for mid-level leadership to read them, process them and then share them with their staffs. Of course implementation needed to occur almost immediately, so little time was allowed for staff to process their loss.

Some mid-level managers started to demonstrate both resistance and ambivalence. They began to question if the new changes were suited to our system. We also began to notice some cracks in Administration, as our CEO became less visible and available for us. We were trying to hold onto some of our worth and value as new leadership styles, personnel changes and a newly introduced culture came rolling our way. We desired to be recognized and accepted for who we were and what we could contribute. No one from corporate ever told us that they appreciated us and what we had done in this market. They did however, mention that they made a bid for our system prior to this one but couldn't work it out at that time. Many procedures changed that staff did not agree with or understand the rationale behind them. Their suggestions on how to improve processes were deflected by the response, "This is what corporate wants," or "This is a new day." When I heard people using phrases such as, "That's not the way we did it before," or openly questioning and challenging new processes and policies, it became clear that they were feeling pushed back into a subjective role that was much different than what they had experienced under Triad.

This is the phase when directors were vying for acknowledgement and their place in this new structure. Mission, vision and value statements changed quickly. A new culture was introduced, but adopting and learning it certainly would take some time. At the writing of this book four years after being acquired by CHS, mid-level managers have participated in nearly 15 Leadership Development Institute initiatives, and we are finally starting to see the results. Our culture is becoming more unified, transparent and observable. Our slow pace in adopting a new culture was due, in part, to rapid changes in staff, leadership, policies and procedures. Obviously, some of this slow pace was due to personal resistance. A new system will not function the same way as the old. The new may be better and more functional or the other way around. Requiring employees to buy into a new culture void of processing their loss is going to slow the process considerably. On the other hand, there were those of us who recognized early on that a culture of care already was in place in the new ownership, for the most part. All we had to do was implement the tools CHS already had developed. This meant less work for us, which resulted in a desire to get it up and going. In the Triad system, we were working hard to create our own culture, since the company was brand new. CHS had Quint Studer's Community Cares culture implemented in its hospitals, and all we needed to do was to get it explained and adopted in ours. As stated earlier, the process of hardwiring many facets of Community Cares has taken us nearly four years. A new Leadership Evaluation Management tool was implemented, to keep track of corporate and department-specific goals. This has helped us increase leadership accountability.

BEHAVIORS:

As the changes began to roll out, it was obvious that some were still reticent, for one reason or another. They have shed their former identity and are taking on a new one, which generates more questions:

- "How will we be treated in this new culture?"
- "What about our benefits? What will they take away?"

By this time, most mid-level managers realized that this sale provided a handsome return to former leadership in the Triad corporation, and we all knew that CHS wouldn't want us if they didn't think that it was a money-making proposition. To get a financial equilibrium established, we knew that cuts would have to be made, and it was not those in CHS's leadership who would make sacrifices – it was our directors and employees who would pay the price for corporate successes. More questions:

- "How will we survive in this new corporation?"

- "How do they do business or is it a new day?"
- "What about Customer Service in this new corporation?"
- "Is this a culture that is patient-centered?"

Insecurities, additional stress and the loss of dreams were being experienced. Cutting staff to adopt a new staffing matrix and realigning our PTO (personal time off) structure were major changes that many struggled through.

PASTORAL FOCUS:

I was visiting with the Auxiliary Director on one of our campuses, and she asked me, "C.J., how do you handle staff members who need to vent as a result of corporate mandates and changes?" I responded by saying, first of all they need someone who is neutral and will listen as they lament about the changes and challenges being experienced. Add to that the challenges staff members are facing at home as a result of a monumental economic downturn, and we have a real opportunity for Pastoral Care. Staff members not only have the pressures of shuffling through corporate changes, there are dynamic changes in the home that they often bring to work with them. While some people will immerse themselves in work to escape the challenges of home, if they come to work and find the same challenges, this compounding situation creates a real morass that can adversely affect morale. It is these individuals who need pastoral presence desperately. It was important for me to remember that people in this phase were not demonstrating a victim mentality but a natural reaction to their changing world of work.

Yxy = Positioning Phase

Coordinate positioning note: The new corporation Y is clearly in control and its Administration is in place. The positioning of the xy is important here. While the y group may be few in number at this time, the x group has given up most, and this fact should be understood and acknowledged by Administration. The former Triad mid-level managers needed acceptance and recognition for what they contributed or brought to the table. It's like athletes moving to a new school and trying out for a sport with a new coach. The athletes want to do their best and make a good impression. It takes a few scrimmages for the team to learn each other's skill levels. The goal is to blend diverse talents together to form a well-functioning team that is capable of winning.

It is in this phase that a CEO must spend time assessing his or her "players" and their strengths and weaknesses; spend money on bringing them together for functions that build team unity; and spend time with them as they learn a new culture. The cost of not doing this is a high one to pay. It will have a direct effect on how quickly they will move through the next phase. Mid-level managers and others will be paying close attention to how lean or top-heavy Administration becomes under a new corporate ownership. There must be a sensitive balance in the eyes of the managers and staff.

Managers who do not maintain the same level of acceptance and positioning may consider leaving. Some mid-level managers found themselves functioning with an old mindset but we were reminded that it was a "new day." Accordingly, the tension between the old way of doing things and the "new day" mindset melted away. Some directors were let go early in the transition process, as consolidation of departments began to occur. Some social work staff did not fit the corporate model of utilizing nurse Case Managers, so they were let go. It was still not quite clear what the corporate model was for some departments. While this phase can become an opportunity to "clean house," some employees who possess desirable skills but who take longer to make adjustments run the risk of being discarded. Along with a new CEO comes another learning curve, and many changes in his or her administrative team.

BEHAVIORS:

An attempt to hang on to their status and positioning in this new environment is the order of business for many mid-level managers. Getting to know the accountability structure and what is expected of the CFO and others is also on the agenda. It is important to remain positive and patient during this phase. Avoid using us vs. them themes because such practices can impede team cohesiveness. When someone resigns or is let go, there always are questions that will go unanswered, and in some cases, no closure can be found. Often, when Administration members or mid-level managers resign or are let go, it is announced with a positive "spin," no matter what the circumstances.

PASTORAL FOCUS:

During this phase I went about emphasizing everyone's importance in fulfilling our mission, vision and values. I "managed up" (spoke positively about) every staff member I could find and also projected a caring attitude. For those who are confident in their skills and abilities, this phase had less of an impact. Being present for those who were obviously struggling to find their place was important to me.

Yyx = Integration/Assimilation/Alignment Phase

Coordinate positioning note: The x employees are learning the leadership and functioning of the Yy system and its structure. They now see how they fit into it. The old identity is dissipating, and new identity is taking shape. CHS and its policies and procedures were now in place, and if we were holding onto anything from Triad, it would be a mere memory. Moving through this phase took some time, but the Community Cares initiative helped us through much of it. It takes time to "break in" a new pair of shoes, even if they are made of the softest leather available. In this phase, I saw that each hospital was beginning to experience some equilibrium again, and managers were becoming more comfortable with how they fit into the new structure. Mid-level managers began aligning their skills and leadership abilities with the new culture. Let me stress that up to this point, it is difficult to experience much cohesiveness among mid-level managers related to a new culture. A new culture is like preparing for a formal event – learning what the event represents, what appropriate attire is expected and showing up is all part of the process. New managers will arrive who are a part of the (Y) domain and they will begin to assess staff. If an employee under their leadership does not align with the model they have been espousing they will begin to reshape their staff accordingly.

BEHAVIORS:

Feelings of acceptance and a more positive attitude return. It is more common to see smiles and laughter as the "swagger" returns. Managers feel more at peace, and their team members pick up on the change. Realizing that our healthcare system was a living organism, powered by relational beings, as opposed to a corporate machine, was important to me. Productivity began to rise as managers got in rhythm with the culture and expectations of Administration. The focus began to shift back on the patient and his or her needs. Managers and staff again realized that it was not about them, but rather the patients and their journeys toward healing and wellness.

PASTORAL FOCUS:

This is the time when affirmation should continue as you notice new energy within management. As noted in the above behavior, staff will recognize this energy and respond to the positive attitude that emanates from their leadership. Always remember that staff cannot rise above their leaders! Managers are there to lead, and their staffs expect no less from.

Yy = Acculturated/Cohesive Phase

Coordinate positioning note: Our corporation and healthcare system owns its own identity and culture. Its mission, vision and values are engrained into its everyday functioning. The employees of the sold entity have done their grief work and accepted the reality of their new environment. They have become members of a new, cohesive team, actively embracing a new culture. Their mantra becomes, "Let's do it," and the momentum begins. Acceptance and a strong sense of belonging take over. HCAHPS scores begin to rise, as the team works together as a cohesive unit. New employees sense the synergy occurring within the hospital or healthcare system, and they desire to contribute. Total acceptance and understanding of a new culture is prevalent. Policies and procedures that enhance functionality and understanding are in place, as things begin to run like a well-oiled machine!

BEHAVIORS:

Before I get too "warm and fuzzy" here, let me point out that this also is the phase when corporations run the risk of functioning merely as an organization and not an organism, made up of people who have minds, bodies and spirits. If sacrifices are made to the "corporate gods" to support a bigger bottom line, without regard for employees' needs to feel rewarded, recognized and valued, the organization likely will not thrive. Profitability will be the focal point, and those rewarded will be those who are the best stewards of this cause. If bonuses are given to some employees and not to others, this can create a chasm. Some will trade their more experienced and well-compensated nurses for those who are younger and less costly – and possibly less effective. "Flex" hours will be the new focus, and personalities will change with the rise and fall of numbers. As barometric pressure impacts behavior, patient census numbers and EBITDA (earnings before interest, taxes, depreciation and amortization) impact staff behavior.

PASTORAL FOCUS:

In this phase, it is incumbent upon Pastoral Care providers to be a present help and balancing entity. Pastoral Care providers must enjoy the moment, along with others and continue to be vigilant about their environment and the ever-developing culture of care. When corporate mandates roll are handed down, stay focused on the human element. Staff come to work each day with myriad personal issues about which you may learn. Being present for them, as well as patients, family members, staff, physicians and Administration is valued presence.

ADDITIONAL COMMENTS:

The manner in which these phases are processed by staff will directly affect the outcome of an acquisition and how quickly that hospital, healthcare system or other corporate entity becomes an acculturated, productive system. The cost of not spending the time, energy, talent and money on bringing your staff through these phases is staggering. We all know that the healthier the staff, the larger the profits and the better care patients will receive. Training employees about these phases in an open manner is highly recommended and will be greatly appreciated. It is my recommendation that a one-day seminar, including "open forum" time, be required. In that format, the leader can lay out the phases that we have just walked through and offer newly acquired employees some information on what the new owners will bring to the table. This process would greatly advance a newly acquired hospital or healthcare system toward acceptance, accountability and cohesiveness. It would also allow a new culture to be integrated much more quickly and get valuable employees re-engaged, with a renewed sense of purpose! Knowing what to expect emotionally, behaviorally and pastorally when you experience the loss of an identity and take on a new one is valuable. My hope is that understanding the process and feeling the presence of Pastoral Care through each phase of it will keep you and your professional skills aligned with compassionate care for those who need it most.

Key Points:

1. Anytime a new hospital is purchased in corporate healthcare, this diagram can be reviewed and used as a primer for administration, mid-level management and staff.

2. Introducing culture change prior to the Integration Phase (Yyx) is almost certain to lead to frustration and elevated turnover.

3. Too much change introduced in the midst of closure work and unresolved grief will overwhelm employees and have a negative impact on their productivity.

4. Allow the process time to work. Not all individuals process loss in the same way or at the same pace.

5. When employees are empowered, they become more engaged in the process, and personal agendas take a back seat.

6. Remain neutral and use appropriate pastoral presence and authority. Pastoral Care providers are an advocate for many in the process.
7. Some CEOs use their faith to model their leadership style and expectations. Don't let this distract from Pastoral Care's professional role.

Chapter Five – Prioritizing Pastoral Care Needs

I would like to spend a few moments to suggest that Administrators, Directors of Pastoral Care and managers/directors to whom Pastoral Care providers report sit down with an inter-disciplinary team to come up with a realistic Priority of Needs list. The purpose of this list is to gain a clear understanding of the type of situation or cases where pastoral presence is absolutely necessary and expected. Don't forget input from the nursing staff, since they are on the front lines of providing care and often know best when to call for Pastoral Care support. Perhaps during National Hospital Week, would be a good time to seek staff input in this area. Creating a list of Pastoral Care needs and asking staff to prioritize them for you would get the ball rolling. This step is crucial and must be completed before a cost-effective Pastoral Care program that works for your hospital or healthcare system can be developed.

Staff should rate the following events that may be likely to require Pastoral Care services. Rate them from one to five, with one being the least important and five being the most important.

Random patient visit   1 2 3 4 5

Physician consult   1 2 3 4 5

Patient death   1 2 3 4 5

Trauma 1		2	3	4	5
Code Blue	1	2	3	4	5
Nursing referral	1	2	3	4	5
Physician referral	1	2	3	4	5
Angry patient	1	2	3	4	5
Advance Directive request	1	2	3	4	5
Administrative request	1	2	3	4	5
Death of staff member	1	2	3	4	5
Education of staff	1	2	3	4	5
Patient leaving AMA (against medical advice)	1	2	3	4	5
Disruptive patient or family member	1	2	3	4	5
Emotional family member	1	2	3	4	5
Local clergy access	1	2	3	4	5

In tallying up the responses, a clear picture will emerge that will serve to guide the development of a Priority of Needs list that can be adopted for a hospital or healthcare system. This list will serve a few important purposes: It will keep Chaplains focused and administration, physicians, directors and nursing staff informed on the type of needs that warrant a "Pastoral Care" page in your organization. This information may be incorporated into the employee orientation process, to ensure that newly hired nurses know under what circumstances they should page Pastoral Care.

Soliciting broad-based input to construct a Priority of Needs list reveals expectations that administration, mid-level managers and staff have of Pastoral Care responses. There may be additional tasks assigned to the Pastoral Services department of which others are unaware. For instance, Pastoral Care Directors may chair or coordinate Biomedical Ethics Committee(s), Institutional Review Boards, Joint Commission RI Chapters, Quality teams, Benevolence Funds, United Way campaigns, Volunteers, etc. It is important as a Director of Pastoral Care to prioritize your department responsibilities so they do not take away from the poignant needs of patients and staff. If staffing is such that Pastoral Care can take on additional tasks such as those listed previously, they will serve to elevate your involvement as an inter-disciplinary team member and take some of the load off other mid-level managers who may be experiencing pressing needs. Don't throw caution to the wind, and remember that Pastoral Care providers need good self-care to keep focused on the delivery of pastoral presence to patients, family, staff and physicians. Pastoral presence does not mean being everywhere and involved in everything.

Another issue related to a Priority of Needs list that I would like to touch on briefly is that sometimes, nurses and volunteers page a Chaplain out of their own need. This occurs more often than one might imagine. Providing care for others can trigger unexpected emotions and behaviors in nurses and other healthcare workers. This is cause for the Chaplain to assess not only the reason for the page but the reason behind the page. In fact, I have received scores of pages that obviously were not about the patient but an SOS plea from a nurse who was attempting to serve a difficult patient or family member. Jay, (not his real name) was a nurse in our Medical Intensive Care Unit and a prime example. When Jay paged, it was usually a "STAT" (urgent) page. Once I arrived, it usually was obvious that Jay was more upset than the patient or family member for whom he was requesting assistance. As it turned out, Jay's wife, also a nurse in our system, was dying of cancer. This was a second marriage for her, and the children from her first marriage were creating issues for both of them. Often, a patient's family dynamics would trigger some of Jay's challenges in his own family system, so he immediately would page the Chaplain. Also, for imminent deaths, he was experiencing anticipatory grief issues and could not handle emotional scenes very well, so he would call us early on. Once I would arrive on the floor, I could see the relief on his face, and he would greet me somewhat emotionally and tell me that he didn't think that it would be too long. Once again, the issue of his wife's impending death was looming heavy for him. Often, a volunteer will see someone crying in the hallway and page a Chaplain to intervene. While that is certainly appropriate, many times, the volunteer's anxiety is much more an issue than the tears of the visitor or family member. We have encouraged our volunteers to suggest a visit to the Chapel for visitors or family members who have a deep need to let their souls weep.

To educate our nurses and other clinical staff on spiritual assessments, I have put together a training module and placed it on the hospital intranet for easy access. Your hospital or healthcare system's Priority of Needs list should be printed and distributed for all staff to see. My suggestion is that the Priority of Needs list be revisited and re-assessed each year, as things change rapidly in healthcare. The Priority of Needs list will help Chaplains prioritize their time, which often is a challenge in a busy hospital or healthcare setting. As each Pastoral Care page is received, there is a need to prioritize it. In supervising students, I have learned that some catch on to prioritizing easily, while others struggle to learn this skill. As students experience multiple CPE units, they eventually get a handle on it.

Running a cost-effective Pastoral Care Department:

During this time of economic downturn, it is time for Pastoral Care departments to work "smarter" than ever before. By doing so, corporate-run hospitals and healthcare systems can continue to provide cost effective pastoral presence and care for those in need. We are at a time when thinking "outside the box" is paramount for survival. That being said, I am not an advocate of CEOs receiving bonuses and salary increases when staff are requested to make cuts in their budgets, eliminating many valuable programs designed to address unique facets of human experience. As studies bear out, the work of a professional Chaplain will have a positive effect on patient satisfaction scores, which, in turn, can affect reimbursement and market share. Taking into consideration educational requirements, Clinical Pastoral Education training, board certification, endorsement and ordination requirements, Chaplains should be compensated accordingly. Another item that I would like to emphasize is the need for continuing education of Chaplains. Most everyone else in healthcare is required to stay current on the latest developments within their respective professions. At many national meetings, I hear the story over and again of many Chaplains having to pay their own way to these training sessions, due to cuts in reimbursement for training and travel. This can place a hardship on many Chaplains and their respective relationships with their cognate group.

After the Priority of Needs assessment is done, the results should be tallied and placed in a hierarchy on a pyramid, as I have done for our healthcare system in the following example.

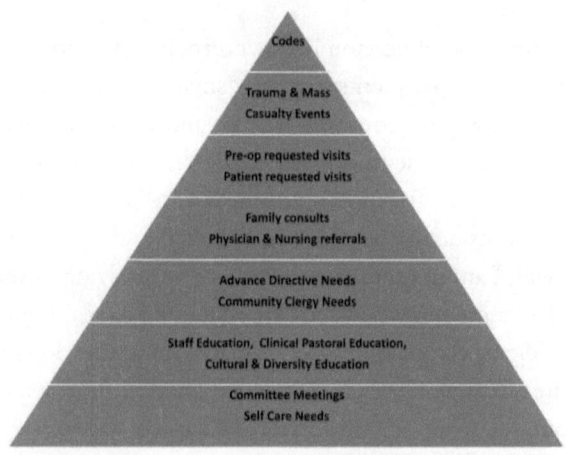

This prioritizing pyramid lists the most important event in the apex. The example I have shared may not fit every hospital or healthcare system, but it may help you do some critical assessment on how you provide prioritized Pastoral Care in your environment. My encouragement is that you take what fits for your own prioritization.

Let's take a few moments to focus on fulfilling Joint Commission's RI standards related to spiritual, religious and cultural needs assessments. The Patient Rights (RI) standards directly state what is required of a hospital or healthcare system in meeting a patient's spiritual, religious and cultural needs. (27) Complying with the Joint Commission Standards is imperative to achieve accreditation. My opinion is that some of the methods used by corporate-run hospitals to accomplish the required assessment do not meet the intent of the standard.

First and foremost, the person performing a patient's spiritual, religious and cultural assessment must be qualified to do so. Directors of Pastoral Care will want to ensure that their staffs are trained and qualified to do that assessment. In fact, every Pastoral Care provider should have the ability to make spiritual assessments trans-culturally and in an inter-faith and age specific manner.

Students enrolled in our CPE program are taught the stages of spiritual development and also are able to demonstrate effective Pastoral Care across the age spectrum. They have received didactic instruction on cultural dynamics and can pick up on a patient's spiritual and religious health. The students and contract Chaplains in our healthcare system are given a basic spiritual assessment tool that they can hardwire into their assessments. When used, it cuts through many layers and creates a starting point for a deeper spiritual assessment and Pastoral Care work. The following five questions help the Pastoral Care provider stay focused on the patient's spiritual Self.

1. Is the patient at peace with God or his or her higher power?

2. Is the patient at peace with the Self?
3. Is the patient at peace with family, staff, physician and others?
4. Is the patient at peace with his or her environment?
5. Is the patient at peace with his or her treatment, diagnosis and/or prognosis?

I am reminded of this five-question approach to a quick spiritual assessment every time I enter a patient's room, raise my hand and say, "Hi." The five fingers on my waving hand represent to me the five-question assessment.

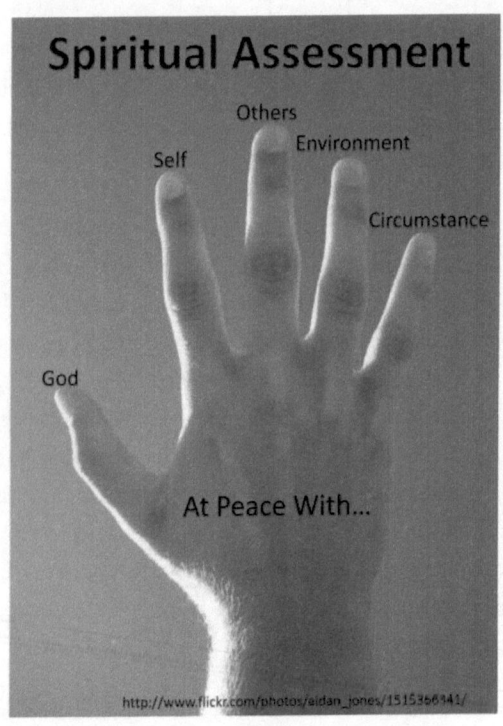

Spiritual Assessment

Others
Environment
Self
Circumstance
God

At Peace With...

http://www.flickr.com/photos/aidan_jones/1515356341/

If there is a "no" response to any of the questions, it is time for me to ask "What's going on?" and take notice of other factors (both verbal and non-verbal) that may be present in the patient. If the patient is stuck in an age-specific development phase, that fact usually is a good indicator of where they need to return for their soul work. The truly spiritual patient is one who is at peace with all the elements listed above. That being said, it does not mean that he or she doesn't have an issue or a story to be told, or that that something isn't stirring the waters of their soul.

Chapter Six – Sustainable Pastoral Presence

Thinking "Outside the Box"

As corporate acquisitions continue to swoop up community and not-for-profit hospitals and healthcare systems throughout America, Directors of Pastoral Care and their departments find themselves being transported from a "hometown U.S.A." atmosphere into a Wall Street dynamic. In order to keep Pastoral Care services present and "sustainable" in this ever-changing healthcare environment, Directors of Pastoral Care must start thinking "outside the box". The challenge is to discover new and cost-effective ways to fulfill the Pastoral Care Priority of Needs in their hospital or healthcare system. If that is not done, and done quickly, Directors of Pastoral Care run the risk of losing valued services. Those directors who can make cost-effective changes in short order certainly will be the ones to find "sustainability" in corporate healthcare.

The following diagram shows several Pastoral Care services that can be found in many hospitals and healthcare system throughout America. It identifies a broad spectrum of services extended to patients, staff, physicians, area clergy and the community. The aforementioned Priority of Needs list for a hospital or healthcare system may serve to challenge administrators and Directors of Pastoral Care to broaden their Pastoral Care services and examine cost-effective ways to deliver these services. A note of caution here: additional services that are added to the Priority of Needs list may require additional man-hours and funding. One thing to keep in mind is that no matter how many services or programs you provide, they can never take the place of the healing that can occur when a patient processes the inner struggles that keep them from connecting to their plan of care. The Chaplain's presence with patients should never be sacrificed to "the program gods." We should not be so naive as to think that there should be a program or support group for every need or that one program can cover them all.

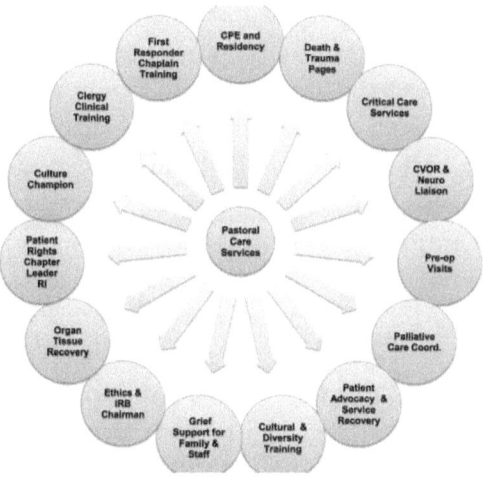

In addition to the programs and services in this graph, Directors of Pastoral Care and their staff members may find themselves doing grand rounds, speaking to community groups, nursing classes, hospice organizations, churches, Stephen Ministry groups or community service organizations. They are apt to speak on issues such as advance directives, death and dying, Allow Natural Death orders, suicide, hope and other specific topics. These are great ways to foster community support and build bridges into your community.

LEAVING THE STATUS QUO

When approached by my boss in 2008 and asked what would happen if we did away with Pastoral Care in our healthcare system, for some reason I never felt an overwhelming sense of panic, but rather a calm assurance that something good was going to come out of this event. The question certainly told me what administration was contemplating. As I processed the question and responded to my boss, there was a calmness and sense of confidence in my reply. First of all, I told him that I certainly didn't want to lose my job, and secondly the community would be "up in arms" if that were to happen. My boss had done his homework by reading local newspaper articles written 12 years prior, when eliminating Pastoral Care in our system was eliminated by Quorum Health Resources as a cost saving measure. Administration at that time experienced intense community criticism when the news broke. It didn't take long for them to reinstate Pastoral Care services, but so much community trust was lost, that it took years for the healthcare system to recover. In retrospect, the event with my boss served to remove me from a status quo existence and projected me into a more creative-thinking mode. I was about to enter some exciting and scary times. While nearby competitor hospitals were adding Pastoral Care staff, we were being asked to eliminate ours. Shortly after that meeting, I realized that it was time to find a way to become sustainable. Experiencing one corporate acquisition after another, along with multiple rounds of staff reductions was enough. We deserved some

138

sustainability! Our patients, staff, physicians and community were truly appreciative of our services, and we knew it. Often it takes being shaken up for a person's creative energy to start flowing – if there is any creativity in the tank at all. There's nothing like the thought of losing one's staff, position and all that you have worked to create to wake you up to a new reality. The two Chaplains in my department were immediately changed to PRN status as a result of our meeting, and they eventually became contract Chaplains when the Institute that was created.

After that meeting, with my free-flowing creative juices flowing wide open, I wasted no time formulating a workable plan. The wheels started turning! The Clinical Pastoral Education program was such a needed resource in our community, and I was going to draw a "line in the sand" on this one. CPE was an educational component of our department, and I knew it was the area where sustainability could begin for us. It was possible to spin it off into a free-standing educational Institute, from which point this new entity could contract with the healthcare system as a clinical site in which students could complete their required clinical time. This would help meet our Pastoral Care coverage needs by allowing CPE interns to respond to the Pastoral Care needs of patients, family members, staff and physicians within our system. This free-standing educational Institute would be a wonderful bridge to our community, focusing on training clergy, seminary students, first-responders and others who were interested in learning the art of Pastoral Care. This step forward meant leaving the security of a traditional healthcare-base. Yes, there were some moments when doubts crept in, but the inner assurance that everything was going to work out kept me focused. We all have heard it said that in challenging times, people start thinking creatively. From my experience, I found truth in that assertion. We are only as limited as we allow ourselves to be. All this positive projection kept me centered on keeping pastoral presence available for those who needed it most.

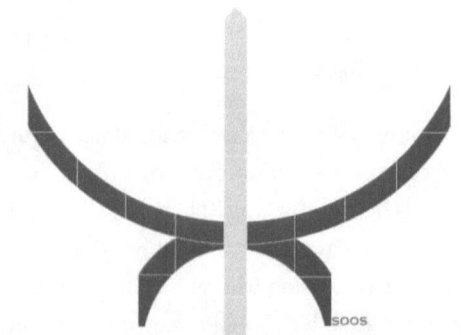

NORTHWEST ARKANSAS
Clinical Pastoral Education Institute

CREATING FREE-STANDING STATUS

Immediate plans were laid down, and I began putting together a proposal (for our COO) that included establishing Northwest Arkansas Clinical Pastoral Education Institute, Inc. This Institute was to be dedicated to teaching the art of Pastoral Care to interested individuals in our community. Our motto is "community-supported community support." This plan would mean immediate financial relief for the healthcare system. Making Pastoral Care sustainable in our healthcare system was off to a good start. As I shared my vision with my boss, I was greatly encouraged by his support of the idea. Together, we presented the proposal to our COO, who immediately endorsed it with great enthusiasm, and a win-win dynamic was born.

The work officially started at that time. Our first order of business was to solicit a board of directors who not only believed in our objective, but who would also work to support its purpose through some challenging times that lay ahead. I knew that we needed a broad spectrum of members on the board, so I invited area clergy, physicians within our healthcare system and my boss to be members. Every person to whom I "pitched" the idea was more than willing to serve. They encouraged and supported the idea of creating sustainability and establishing an Institute that would be focused on Clinical Pastoral Education. Our first order of business was to file articles of incorporation with the state of Arkansas. A local attorney who had done work for our hospital in the past graciously agreed to do the filing of our incorporation papers for a nominal fee. We then needed to file our 501(c)(3) non-profit status with the IRS. This was a crucial step in order for us to receive grants and donations for the Institute. The University of Arkansas School of Law's Legal Clinic is nearby, so we solicited their help in filing our IRS tax-exempt application and associated forms. The University of Arkansas Legal Clinic (28) provides senior law students the opportunity to gain basic competencies in specific areas of practice commonly encountered by entry-level lawyers. Within eight months from the time we filed our 501(c)(3) application, we received a letter of determination from the IRS that we were considered a tax-exempt entity. That was truly an exciting day and I began writing grant applications immediately. Tuition that students had paid for their CPE in 2008 was reimbursed to the Institute by the healthcare system, and those funds served to get us started. We knew that there would be additional tuition funds coming from enrolling students that could be used to pay contract Chaplains who would cover Pastoral Care pages when students were not on call. Our department also contracted to provide Pastoral Care Services to an in-house Long Term Acute Care (LTAC) hospital that rented a floor in our hospital, and that, too, provided some revenue for the Institute. Revenue from student tuition fees helped some and we also offered students an opportunity to pay for their tuition through work-study. They would sign up for additional call shifts and receive credit toward their tuition. The greater the number of students enrolled in the program, and the more work-study hours interns were willing to provide, the greater the distance we would cover on a 24/7 coverage schedule, and the less we would have to pay for contract Chaplains. The board of directors and I knew that the Institute would have future opportunities to contract with other entities in our area for Pastoral Care coverage. This also would open up placement options for CPE students we were training at the Institute.

We all knew that there were many educational options that the Institute could offer in addition to a Clinical Pastoral Education program to area clergy, seminary students, spiritual leaders and others interested in enhancing their skills in Pastoral Care. One of our first priorities was to create an annual Pastoral Care seminar for area clergy, offering them an opportunity to hear from a national leader in the Pastoral Care movement on a cutting-edge Pastoral Care topic. Our first speaker in 2010 was Robert C. Dykstra, who spoke on the subject of "Hope, in a Seemingly Hopeless Situation." More than 125 clergy, Chaplains, physicians, social workers and counselors attended from our area. The seminar was underwritten by the Northwest Medical Center – Springdale Auxiliary. We set up tables in the foyer for organizations that wanted to share information about their products and services with our audience. Another education opportunity that we are still working on is the training of First-responder Chaplains, who, so often, are chosen from among their ranks simply because they are the most religious person on the team. It is also our goal to provide a Clergy Clinical Week to familiarize area clergy with the Healthcare environment and our hospital setting. The hospital can be an intimidating environment for them and helping them experience our interdisciplinary functioning would indeed be helpful. Ultimately, as funds become available, the Institute would like to establish a residency program for CPE students that qualify for a "fast track" to Chaplaincy certification. These programs are high on our priority list and continue to be communicated on a regular basis to the Institute's board of directors and projected to all the philanthropic individuals and foundations with whom we communicate, in our quest for funding.

While CPE interns are on call for the Institute, they are involved in providing random pastoral visits, responding to pages for Pastoral Care and providing liaison service between the Cardiovascular Operating Room (CVOR) team and family members in the reception areas. They are also present for staff and physicians within Northwest Health System. When CPE interns are not scheduled for their clinical time, the Institute uses contract Chaplains (former

CPE students) and pays them an hourly rate for carrying the pager and a set hourly fee for responding in person to pages requiring pastoral presence. This is where establishing a Priority of Needs list has helped us keep costs under control. The funds generated by student tuition, grants, fund-raisers and other donations are used to compensate contract Chaplains.

As the Institute began to find its footing, I became keenly aware of my coalescing roles. As I pause to reflect on this journey and recommend it as a possible course for other Pastoral Care departments, I am acutely aware that it takes knowing and being connected to your community in special ways and the personal ability to creatively function on many levels to make it work. What I discovered is that there is room to grow a solid CPE program that trains individuals in the art of Pastoral Care, as long as the community is willing to support it. It takes a Director of Pastoral Care and a good board of directors who can catch a vision and can put a lot of pieces together.

In this economic downturn that has gripped our nation, I realize that hospitals and healthcare system funds may not be as readily available to set up this type of Pastoral Care program. Timing is of the essence as well. Here in Northwest Arkansas, we have been insulated, to some degree, from the deep economic downturn. Much of this "insulation" is due in large part to major corporations, such as Wal-Mart Stores Inc., Tyson Foods and J.B. Hunt Transport that are headquartered here. We also have had extremely positive population growth over the last decade, which is reflected in our 2010 Census figures. Those areas in our nation who have experienced drastic losses, I believe still can find some creative ways to obtain funding. The following are just a few options, but most of the time, securing funding simply boils down to getting the word to the right people in your community. A good piece of advice that I continue to hear from great fund-raisers is that people give to people. Here's some food for thought:

•GRANTS: There are many foundations locally and nationally from which to request funding. While it can be discouraging when grant applications are denied, remember that foundations have money to give, and Pastoral Care programs and services can help them put it to good use. Convincing a foundation of your worthiness takes time and good writing skills. Working the grant system effectively is a bit like panning for gold. Be strategic and follow the application procedure carefully. Finding gold involves finding a good stream and a great deal of sifting. The more sifting you do, the greater your chances of finding nuggets. Look in places where gold is likely to be, where conditions are favorable. Look for a good grant writer who has the drive and patience to work the process properly. Grants will invariably be denied, but stay focused and keep them in front of foundation boards.

•DESIGNATED CHARITABLE GIVING: Pastoral Care Directors might be surprised at how many physicians, staff and others in the community want to support pastoral presence but simply have not been asked to do so. Helping people through times of crisis has a positive effect on a community's well-being. There are many people who would enjoy teaming up with such a noble cause as Chaplaincy. As a 501(c)(3) entity, a Pastoral Care program can provide charitable donation receipts to contributors who may need that for tax purposes. They can deduct their giving to the extent allowable by law.

•**CHURCHES/DENOMINATIONS**: Area clergy benefit from having pastoral presence available in a medical center or healthcare system. Not only does our Institute provide educational opportunities for them, we are present for their members who work in our system. Our Pastoral Care providers are also present for clergy when they lose a parishioner and need pastoral presence themselves. When clergy are out of town or unaware that one of their parishioners has been admitted to the hospital, they appreciate the fact that a Pastoral Care provider is present in the hospital for those parishioners to call upon. CPE students at the Institute are reminded that just because a pastor is present for a trauma or death of one of their members or our patients, it doesn't mean that their services aren't needed. If a local clergy person has a small congregation, he or she may be just as impacted by the event as the immediate family. Pastors can have a strong influence on their outreach committees, so when it comes to supporting pastoral presence in a local medical center or healthcare system, they should be visited personally.

•**ENDOWMENT FUNDS**: This type of funding takes a lot of work and some substantial contributions to get started but it is an excellent way to help create sustainability for Pastoral Care programs. It usually begins with the generous contribution from someone very close to Pastoral Care in your hospital or system. Creating an endowment fund provides continued financial resources for a Pastoral Care department, and a good financial adviser always is recommended to keep it on track.

•**FUND-RAISING EVENTS**: This funding option also takes a good deal of work, but it can be very fun and financially rewarding. This is an area where creativity can run wild, and activities can range from banquets with specific themes to fun events for the community and everything in-between. Since we have many avid golfers in our area, the thought of hosting a golf invitational seemed logical for us. Knowing that we had several physicians who were avid golfers, too, we settled on naming it the "Physician SpecialTee Golf Invitational." Our focus was to reach out to specialty medical practices in the community and have them support a worthy cause. No matter if they were Podiatrists, Nephrologists, Immunologists, Psychologists or any other variety of medical specialist, we wanted them to partner with us. Our hospital vendors and community businesses were very helpful in providing support for this cause.

•**ANNUAL FINANCIAL CAMPAIGN**: Early one morning, I met with Jim Johnson at Panera Bread in Fayetteville, Ark. Jim is an insightful man who, at the writing of this book, is in the midst of raising $50 million to build a U.S. Marshals Museum just 70 miles down the road in Fort Smith, Ark. At first, my thought was that Jim would not want to waste his time on our small Institute, but I later discovered that he had a unique affinity for compassionate care. Not only did he have experience with the funeral home industry, during time in the military, Jim would knock on the doors of military family members who had lost loved ones.

He also has helped churches in financial campaigns and was willing to work with our board of directors (pro bono) to establish an annual campaign. He knows the power of well-run annual campaigns like that of Father Flanagan's Boys Town. This time, Jim came to us bearing some good news! What a "heavensend." If the Salvation Army can run a campaign to raise thousands upon thousands of dollars, I would think that an Institute providing pastoral presence for the hurting souls of our community could do the same. Perhaps attending one of their training seminars on how to do it would be beneficial.

Moving from a traditional Pastoral Care department to having a department and Institute working hand-in-hand has required an abundance of creative energy and administrative savvy. Moving away from long-standing expectations of a Pastoral Care department and into a new paradigm of Pastoral Care that is driven by prioritized needs will take time to adjust to, so be patient with the process.

OUT-SOURCING PASTORAL CARE

It is obvious that my being an Executive Director of the Institute, Director of Pastoral Care for our healthcare system and CPE supervisor of Pastoral Care interns affords me some exclusive privileges and opportunities that others may not have. There are a few incorporated entities across America whose purpose is to provide trained, certified Chaplains and place them in medical centers, healthcare systems, hospice organizations, industry and other community organizations that may need Pastoral Care presence. While they normally are found in large metropolitan areas, they also can be effective in rural areas that have high concentrations of healthcare needs and services. Some healthcare systems and medical centers that utilize such a service may have their own Director of Pastoral Care or Cultural Diversity Director on staff who contracts with such entities to serve their Pastoral Care coverage needs. In some cases, hospitals or healthcare systems will use the contracted services exclusively. In those cases, the Executive Director will need to market and service those accounts personally. Establishing the Priority of Needs for contracted entities is essential in setting good boundaries.

The incorporated entity gathers Pastoral Care providers and contractually links them up with medical centers, healthcare systems, hospice organizations, nursing homes, industry or other entities interested in paying for someone to cover their Pastoral Care needs. As stated earlier, many industrial and food-service corporations are now utilizing Chaplains as their Employee Assistance Program. Having that personal contact with a Chaplain is a valued asset to their employees and enhances trust and productivity.

With any contract, the devil is in the details. Writing contracts and servicing the needs of the contracted entity is an ongoing administrative responsibility. The executive director of an entity that provides Pastoral Care coverage on this scale is a busy person and will need a good staff and board of directors to help direct its mission and purpose. Not only does such an entity service the contract, they will need to service the needs of the Pastoral Care providers, as well.

In retrospect, one can find meaning and purpose in many events of life. As stated in the beginning pages, my passion was to make quality Pastoral Care presence sustainable, and I was willing to rise to the challenge and think "outside the box" to achieve that objective. As T.S. Eliot said, "God exults when a [person] comes through with a wish of his own." (29) Lewis B. Smedes also said, "Desire adds imagination to our wills and heat to our intentions." (30) Pastoral Care Directors who are filled with passion for their programs but are experiencing some of the corporate trends mentioned earlier should start thinking "outside the box." Don't just lie down and let someone run over you.

Following are some of our current projected programs being offered or awaiting funding at the Northwest Arkansas Clinical Pastoral Education Institute:

•CPE Residency Program

This program would provide CPE interns who qualify with a "fast-track" opportunity to become a board-certified Chaplain.

•CVOR Liaison Service

During open heart cases in our healthcare system, family members receive progress updates from CPE students and/or contract Chaplains. These reports keep family members informed at all times. This service is deeply appreciated by family members and lowers anxiety levels for loved ones.

•First -responder "Chaplain" Training Program

This program will allow the Institute to train 30 area First-responders who function as "Chaplain" for their response team. Each Chaplain will receive 400 hours of supervised training of which one hundred hours will be in didactic sessions. This training is equivalent to one unit of Clinical Pastoral Education.

•Clergy Clinical Week

This is an intensive week of didactics and practical interaction within the clinical environment for area clergy. This program will allow up to forty area clergy from various faith perspectives to spend an intensive week in the clinical environment learning the art of Pastoral Care. This training will assist pastors and spiritual care leaders to be more "pastoral" to patients and family members who are experiencing a crisis due to major trauma, suicide, stroke, mental-health struggles, or other major, grief-producing events. It familiarizes local clergy with the inter-disciplinary approach to care.

•Clinical Pastoral Education

Extended units are offered to seminary students, clergy, spiritual care leaders and others desiring to enhance their Pastoral Care skills.

•Pastoral Care Seminar

A nationally renowned speaker presents on the subject of Pastoral Care to honor physicians, clergy, counselors and Chaplains in our area who give of themselves to help others. CEUs are offered for continuing education purposes.

Chapter Seven – Directors of Pastoral Care & CEOs

My hope is that this book will encourage and challenge Directors of Pastoral Care and their departments to work smarter, be more observant, and provide cost-effective Pastoral Presence and Care to those in need within your hospital or healthcare system. Throughout this book, an attempt has also been made to illustrate the effectiveness of Pastoral Care presence to those who really need to know. In this chapter, I would like to address the role of a Pastoral Care director at the corporate level, specific issues for Directors of Pastoral Care at the local level and then add a few comments for CEOs to consider as they interact with and utilize Pastoral Care providers on all levels.

CORPORATE DIRECTOR OF PASTORAL CARE

In corporations or alliances that own several hospitals in a specific region, or for those larger corporations that are divided into regions or divisions, my suggestion is that a Corporate Director of Pastoral Care & Spiritual Services be hired to oversees Pastoral Care programs throughout the organization to ensure consistency, cost-effective operations, compliance with Joint Commission standards related to patient rights and designing way in which Pastoral Care and presence can interface with HCAHPS functioning. Corporate healthcare systems and alliances would benefit from a cohesive model of Pastoral Care for each medical center to follow. The Corporate Director would develop consistent policies and procedures to best serve corporate objectives and core human needs in the local healthcare setting. A Corporate Director also would help to restructure embedded and often ineffective models of Pastoral Care and certain pastoral staff that may stymie others from thinking "outside the box." As stated previously, some directors and Chaplains may not be the right fit for the hospital or system as it grows, takes on new challenges and expands services. This issue should be pointedly addressed during and after acquisitions. The corporate director of Pastoral Care would ensure that each Director of Pastoral Care and his or her department mirror their community in terms of faith group representation, religious institutions, spiritual and culture sensitivity. Specific training relevant to corporate Pastoral Care initiatives could roll out more effectively for this structure.

While learning the art of Pastoral Care through Clinical Pastoral Education in a clinical setting is the gateway for Pastoral Care providers to be hired in healthcare, those desiring to become Directors of Pastoral Care in corporate healthcare will need specialized training and mentoring. Those desiring to become CEOs, CFOs and CNOs in many healthcare corporations are placed in a two-year program to learn the system and its processes. In addition to CPE and CPE Supervision, perhaps there is room in the Clinical Pastoral Education venue for such a corporate Pastoral Care mentoring model. The Pastoral Care Director must, however, "hit the ground running" and be able to provide services that will impact HCAHPS scores and immediately add to the bottom line in a corporate system. In many faith-based hospitals, one can find a corporate Vice President of Missions, who oversees and mentors to some degree the Director of Missions in local settings. Until his recent death, Foy Ritchie, a leading Pastoral Care educator, was instrumental in championing deeper support and understanding of Pastoral Care in corporate settings. (31)

PASTRORAL CARE DIRECTORS IN HOSPITALS & HEALTHCARE SYSTEMS

A Director of Pastoral Care, who is sure to experience sustainability in corporate healthcare now and into the future, should be well-rounded, flexible, certified and professionally licensed in billable areas. Pastoral Care Directors should be qualified to train medical staff, physicians and community leaders on their respective competency levels. They will also need to be excellent relational beings, inter-disciplinary team members, knowledgeable about corporate systems, well-versed in systems convergence and able to lead effectively through culture and diversity transformations, acquisitions and other healthcare challenges and changes. The successful Pastoral Care Director may even wear a new title, as the scope of services offered by his or her department broadens. In addition, Pastoral Care Directors will need staff or contract Chaplains who are able to put theory and practice together (praxis) into meaningful action that will satisfy corporate objectives and Joint Commission standards as well as meeting the human needs of their hospital or healthcare system in caring, compassionate ways.

In protecting the heritage and legacy of many Directors of Pastoral Care who have served before us, current Directors of Pastoral Care must shoulder some responsibility. Not only must we be vigilant about our environment, we also should supply sensitive, professionally trained Pastoral Care providers who have had Clinical Pastoral Education, cultural and religious sensitivity training, crisis intervention, mass casualty preparedness, cultural diversity education, biomedical ethics training, family systems theory and experience at developing good pastoral presence. Directors of Pastoral Care must take an active role in fulfilling the Joint Commission RI standards in assessing the spiritual and cultural needs of patients and more closely monitor those critical cases that physicians and nurses struggle with on a daily basis. The challenge is to work "smarter" and find creative ways to maintain sustainability for a profession that so many of us have grown to love.

If a hospital or healthcare system is top-heavy with Pastoral Care, the Director of Pastoral Care may find himself or herself fighting to keep it that way. Doing a Priority of Needs assessment may help balance the team, but it's always best to be proactive in getting ahead of the adjustment phases that are sure to come. When the next executive announces that Pastoral Care must be cut, it will help to have a contingency plan ready. Even though Chaplain/patient ratios are projected by professional Chaplain certification groups, (32) such a level of staffing may be impractical in today's corporate environment. So, thinking "outside the box" can make it possible for you to create savings and still provide effective Pastoral Care and presence. At the end of the day, the hospital or health system hopefully will have a balanced Pastoral Care approach that works effectively at fulfilling prioritized needs in a cost-saving manner. If the Pastoral Care team becomes a valued part of inter-disciplinary teams, supporting the mission, vision and values of your organization, while also delivering quality care, it will be a positive reflection on the department's leadership and a wonderful testament to the value Pastoral Care presence brings to many lives.

CEOs

I would be remiss if I did not also offer some reflection and encouragement to CEOs, who control the presence of Pastoral Care in their hospitals and healthcare systems. We all are in this together. Not only are we serving patients, family members, staff and physicians, we are serving community after community all across America and beyond. In my opinion, there is no faster way to raise a community's level of trust in a hospital or healthcare system than to offer a competent, cutting edge medical staff, good HCAHPS scores, specialized services and quality pastoral presence to those who are hurting.

While we all recognize the impact of challenging economic times, it is alarming to observe more and more hospital Pastoral Care departments being squeezed year after year to support a more profitable bottom line. When this happens, valuable services that reach to the core of human need evaporate from the places that need them most. In healthcare centers where Pastoral Care services are no longer available, those in other professions, such as physicians, nurses, Case Managers and administrators themselves are doing their best to be present for those in spiritual and emotional pain. Most do not have professional training or skills in the areas of family systems, crisis and grief support, personality assessments and all the other skills needed to be effectively present for those experiencing times of great stress. These well-meaning healthcare professionals simply are not equipped to do what a professionally trained Pastoral Care provider do. As we have stated previously, people who attempt to minister to these populations without the benefit of proper clinical pastoral training often find that their own pain and unresolved issues are triggered by the distress of the very people they are attempting to help. The end result of being pulled back into their own emotional processing can drain them of professional focus. Working as an inter-disciplinary team is becoming more and more challenging these days, but the fact remains that healthcare will always require a number of professions to work together for the common good – the whole is greater than the sum total of its parts. As a Pastoral Care provider, I have my area of focus, and I'm not going to be doing what a physician or CEO is hired to do. I will support them and "manage them up," but I cannot do their jobs and mine too.

Recently, one of our emergency departments in our health system began using a nurse Case Manager to escort family members to a consultation room and keep them updated during trauma and death. This strategy was an attempt to keep response times low and keep HCAHPS scores up. While the intent was noble, and the Case Manager was diligent in being available and as compassionate as she could be, I knew that she was way out of her "comfort zone." During evening hours and on weekends, our contract Chaplains require an average of 20-30 minutes to arrive when called in, usually because they are not paged as quickly as they should be and because they are on call for all three of our hospitals. On one Monday afternoon, a 3-year-old child was brought into the ED by EMS personnel, with the father in tow. The father was taken to the ED consult room by the nurse Case Manager, and because he was experiencing anticipatory grief, the distraught dad lashed out and hit the wall with his fist, breaking a bone in his hand. This event, while commonly understood by professionally trained Pastoral Care providers, was not handled well by the Case Manager. She was certain that this grieving father was going to hit her, and she fled in terror requesting the unit secretary to call a Chaplain to take over. The child died, and I continued to be present for the parents in that horrible time of loss. Their immediate family was six hours away, and they had no local support system. I was present and helped to get the father's hand tended to by our ED staff. This couple had just experienced a parent's worst nightmare and needed pastoral presence during their time of processing that deep pain. There are no substitutes for professional pastoral presence when it is needed.

Many CEOs and administrators with whom I visit acknowledge the benefits of Pastoral Care services and presence during such cases, but severe cuts and elimination of services still occur. So, what is the disconnect? When confronted with cutting or eliminating Pastoral Care, do the work of assessing Pastoral Care's effectiveness in your hospital or healthcare system. Talk to nurses on acute-care nursing floors and in critical-care areas. Talk with your physicians and ancillary staff as to the real and perceived Pastoral Care needs, and listen to responses from their perspectives. This may include having an outside consultant come and do that assessment for you. Vision doesn't always happen from within. An outside perspective often can spark introspection and provide the impetus for change.

As a Department Director and Executive Director of a Clinical Pastoral Education Training Institute, I know how important it is for the right Pastoral Care person to be placed in the right setting. A skilled and experienced director of Pastoral Care will be able to make those assignments or reassignments as needed to ensure the right fit. In every hospital or healthcare system, there are skilled professionals who have strong personalities and who interact in a highly charged environment, creating opportunities for clashes and confrontations. Pastoral Care providers can be valued inter-disciplinary team members who have a calming effect and help all involved staff focus on their professional purpose: to provide quality and compassionate healthcare for patients. After all, that is what we are all here for, isn't it? Pastoral Care personnel should be valued supporters of the mission, vision, values and culture of the organization as well. If this is not happening, then this is something the Director of Pastoral Care needs to know. If it is the Director of Pastoral Care who is not supportive of the vital elements of the organization's focus, a change in leadership is needed. Once again, doing a Priority of Needs assessment certainly will help any CEO understand how Pastoral Care should function in their setting.

In healthcare, most everyone has an opinion on religion and spirituality that encompasses all world religions and many variant belief systems, as well. Everyone has some kind of idea what Pastoral Care should look like, too. While compassionate employees are a cultural element that effect patient scores, it is appropriately dispensed compassion and accurately directed passion that makes the difference. While a CEO may project values and faith through his or her position, he or she cannot be present for all the spiritual and emotional needs that exist within a hospital or healthcare system. We really do need each other. A CEO who projects a particular brand of religion or too much religious fervor into his or her role runs the risk of blurring the lines and losing the confidence of staff. How so? This goes back to "wearing too many hats." which certainly can diminish professional effectiveness and create "role confusion." A CEO's personal religious commitment is no substitute for professionally delivered Pastoral Care.

In his initial speech to our directors and supervisors, one of our recent CEOs talked about "doing good" as the mantra for his leadership style and what he desired in hospital leadership and staff. It sounded like a sermon, with an invitation at the end for all of us to join him at the front and align ourselves with a higher calling. No matter how tempting it may be for a CEO to project religious beliefs upon others, my encouragement is to embed personal faith into leadership style and search for creative, cost-effective ways to care for the staff and show them your appreciation. Living out faith in this manner is far more effective, and the team will not feel as threatened by such faith statements, which may not sync with their personal beliefs. There always will be tough leadership decisions, so a CEO's record as a compassionate leader will be revealed over time. However, a CEO's testimonial on how faith has sustained him or her in challenging moments at the helm certainly can be effective, when fitly and aptly spoken.

Another of our CEOs (we have had seven in the past 11 years) informed me shortly after his arrival that in his previous hospital, every Friday a 7:30 a.m., he would be available for prayer time in the Board Room. His Director of Pastoral Care, members of his leadership team and some physicians participated. At his request, we instituted that practice in our system. It went on for nearly a year, and often, there were only three or four of us present. We would take turns sharing pressing issues from our respective areas and any personal or professional challenges we may have been experiencing at that time. The sharing would end, followed by a "round-robin" style of group prayer. This became a refreshing time for me and a time of accountability for our small group, but I could tell that it was more exclusive than inclusive. Many felt uncomfortable with the evangelical thrust that permeated the practice.

While some CEOs leave the spiritual care of staff and patients to the Pastoral Care providers they employ, others will take on the role of spiritual leader. A major concern is instances in which CEOs take on this role but know very little about their Pastoral Care team and how much they contribute to quality care and the "bottom line." On the other hand, there are those CEOs who know and appreciate Pastoral Care professionals and honor their presence. The CEO's knowledge regarding Pastoral Care is critical if he or she is to make decisions regarding Pastoral Care services. I encourage all CEOs to get to know their Directors of Pastoral Care well.

Over the years, I have observed some compassionate CEOs and administrators getting so caught up in running hospitals and responding to directives from the corporate headquarters that they lose sight of their team. When this happens, the synergy they once enjoyed begins to wane. Administrators who are mere conduits of higher corporate leadership forfeit their ability to empower those they are chosen to lead. If mid-level managers and directors are not empowered, their creativity is stymied and production certainly will be effected. Empowering directors and mid-level managers to utilize their professional skills will take your team to new heights.

As HCAHPS scores begin to affect reimbursements, pastoral presence can go a long way in raising those scores and keeping them consistent. With reimbursement for services being more and more driven by those satisfaction scores, hospitals and healthcare systems need creative cutting edge thinking that is based on some sound foundational and relational principles that have proven to work. When healthcare professionals view patients as relational beings and empower them to tell their stories, we will begin to see a major shift in our healthcare endeavors. We humans are relational beings, and we really do need each other. Patients who are in pain will always benefit from those who are willing to take time to listen and be present as they process what is churning inside them.

A former Chief Operating Officer in our health system said that if he were a patient in the hospital, he would expect his minister to visit him. When the option to leave Pastoral Care up to the patient's clergy becomes the rationale for eliminating or scaling back Pastoral Care services, it's important to know that a growing number of people throughout America have no church affinity. In George Barna's book, "Grow Your Church from the Outside," he states that the un-churched population in the United States exceeds 100 million. He goes on to say that many more are attending church intermittently, but not on a regular basis. He said, "the numbers consistently point out that those who live without a regular face-to-face faith connection tend to be relatively isolated from the mainstream of society, tend to be non-committal in institutional and personal relationships, and typically revel in their independence." (33) These un-churched and intermittent attendees in America are being admitted to hospitals at the same rate as others, and they have no clergy person to contact. While they state that they do not need Pastoral Care, they certainly would benefit in many ways from the empowerment given them by a professional Pastoral Care provider.

There are many large "mega-churches" across America, in which attendees can get "lost" in their immensity. Church-goers who have sporadic attendance habits may be overlooked altogether. Frequently, pastors call me to let me know they will be out of town for a while, and if any of their congregants are hospitalized, they would appreciate Pastoral Care staff looking in on them. No one calls for the un-churched. When community pastors respond to death and trauma in our system, I encourage our Chaplains to be present as well, because a pastor's reaction to the trauma is not always easy to forecast. We do not relinquish our professional approach to local clergy, and we often discover that clergy need a Chaplain themselves. On another level, I have visited with many of our patients who have asked me not to contact their local pastor for fear that he or she would put their personal information out on the "prayer chain" list or print it in the church bulletin, allowing everyone in the congregation or parish to know. Some patients do not want their pastors to know that they are in the hospital, so that he or she will not be distracted from more pressing pastoral duties. Who is available to provide pastoral presence to these people? Having Pastoral Care presence "manages up" your medical center or healthcare system in the minds of local clergy and other community leaders.

Often, corporations bring in outside CEOs, who have no knowledge of the religious makeup of a community. A new CEO coming on board will make Pastoral Care wonder whether the change in leadership will affect their positions. Even with average CEO tenures ranging between two years and five years, that can be a long time to "muddle through" without Pastoral Care services. Corporations that shuffle CEOs around geographically must remember that each geographical location has its own unique religious and spiritual culture. Here in Northwest Arkansas, our employees have seen Wal-Mart, Tyson Foods, J.B. Hunt and many major corporations function effectively for a very long time. The employees of our healthcare system are vocal about major change, and that can be a challenge for some administrators. However, it is vital for employees to have a voice and for administration to listen. Ultimately, it is administration's decision that everyone will need to respect. That does not mean Administration will get it right all the time. Northwest Arkansas has an abundance of churches, and many observers have said this region is in the "buckle" of the "Bible belt." CEOs need to be aware of this religious dynamic as they interact with community leaders and other constituents.

CONCLUSION

My hope and expectation for Pastoral Care providers in corporate healthcare is that they find the strength and creative ability to move beyond the rhetoric and concerns related to healthcare changes and stay focused on creative ways to be present for patients who are journeying through the healing process. I also hope that Directors of Pastoral Care departments will continue to establish a valuable rapport with CEOs and their administrative teams as they advocate for patients, family members, staff, physicians and others in the community. In order to make pastoral presence sustainable in corporate healthcare, we as Pastoral Care providers will need to sharpen our sense of duty and creativity. We certainly are living in a new day and time, in which pastoral presence can be of even greater value than before. Seize the moment.

Endnotes

Chapter 1

1. Robert C. Dykstra, Pastoral Care Seminar, Oct. 26, 2009, Northwest Arkansas Clinical Pastoral Education Institute, Springdale, AR "quote"

2. PHG Foundation, National Children's Study expanded by Simon Leese, 5 October 2010. www.phgfoundation.org/news/5721

3. Overstreet, Walter E., Coppage/Coppedge Chronicle II 1542-1998 Devon, PA., Cooke Publishing Company. PP 7&8

Chapter 2

4. "Contract Pastoral Care and Education: The Trend of the Future?" VendeCreek, Larry, The Haworth Press, Inc., 1999 p1

5. "Hardwiring Excellence: Purpose, Worthwhile Work, Making a Difference" by Quint Studer , Fire Starter Publishing, Gulf Breeze, FL. 2004 p 117-119

6. The HCAHPS (Hospital Consumer Assessment of Healthcare Providers and Systems) https://www.cms.gov/hospitalqualityinits/30_hospitalhcahp s.asp

7. "Economic Impact Report" - American Hospital Association, Fall of 2010.

8. "Staffing for Quality Chaplaincy Care Services, A Position Paper of the APC Commission on Quality in Pastoral Services," October 1, 2009 Joint Commission

9. "Common Standards for Professional Chaplaincy," Association of Clinical Pastoral Education; Standards and Professional Competencies, College of Pastoral Supervision & Psychotherapy.

10. ibid 4, p 49-58

11. "Developing a culturally competent workforce: A diversity program in progress," Mott, William J. Jr., Journal of Healthcare Management Date: Monday, September 1, 2003

12. 2010 Official Census STATS, Arkansas, Benton & Washington Counties.

Chapter 3

13. "A Pretty Good Person What it Takes to Live with Courage, Gratitude, & Integrity or When Pretty Good Is as Good as You Can Be," Harper, 1990 p 23

14. Carol Taylor in the Supportive Voice Vol. 11 No. 2 in the Summer of 2006

15. Henri J.M. Nouwen Quote

16. ibid 5, p 94

17. "The Empowered Patient: How to Get the Right Diagnosis, Buy the Cheapest Drugs, Beat Your Insurance Company, and Get the Best Medical Care Every Time." Elizabeth Cohen, Ballantine Books, New York, 2010

18. Joint Commission Journal on Quality and Safety, December 2003, Patient centeredness – Addressing Patients' Emotional and Spiritual Needs.

19. "Allow Natural Death--An Alternative To DNR?" by Reverend Chuck Meyer

20. ibid 5, 94

21. Bruss, Jon., "The Circle of Care, Professional Chaplains integral to organization mission" by Rita Kaufman CAE, Association of Professional Chaplain web page, 2010

Chapter 4

22. Weekly Corporate Growth Report, October 30th edition.

23. MarketWatch, March 19, 2007 edition

24. Foa, E., Rothbaum, B., & Furr, J. (2003). "Augmenting exposure therapy with other CBT procedures." Psychiatric Annals, 33(1), 47–56.

25. Abramowitz, J. S. & Kalsy. S. A. (2001) "Recent Developments in the Cognitive-Behavioral Treatment of

Obsessive-Compulsive Disorder." The Behavior Analyst Today, 2 (2), 141–146

26. Rachman, S (1997). "The evolution of cognitive behaviour therapy". In Clark, D, Fairburn, CG & Gelder, MG. "Science and Practice of Cognitive Behaviour Therapy." Oxford: Oxford University Press. pp. 1–26.

Chapter 5

27. Joint Commission Standards, "Comprehensive Accreditation Manual for Hospitals: (CAMH)" © 2008, Pre-publication Version, Joint Commission Resources, Inc., Rights And Responsibility of The Individual RI.01.01.01

Chapter 6

28. University of Arkansas Legal Clinic
http://www.uacted.uark.edu/legalesource/resources.html

29. T. S. Eliot

30. Lewis B. Smedes

Chapter 7

31. ibid 4, p81-85

32. Chaplaincy Today, Volume 21 Number 1, Spring/Summer 2005

33. George Barna, "New Statistics on Church Attendance and Avoidance," March 3, 2008